THIS BOOK

BELONGS TO

....

....

....

Table of Contents

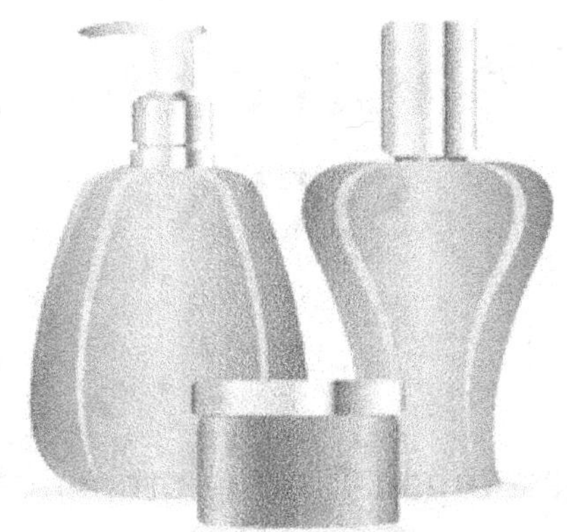

Chapter One:
SKIN

Your skin is your biggest organ. Taking proper care of it can make you look younger, healthier, and give you the extra "it" factor. Dry, sun-damaged skin not taken care of will add years to your appearance. Which nobody wants. Models make it their number one priority to have beautiful, glowing skin and so should you. The three major ways to slow down the process of aging and ensure youthful skin is by using sunscreen, eating healthy, and not smoking. Here are a few of my favorite tips to give me the extra freshness for great looking skin. Enjoy.

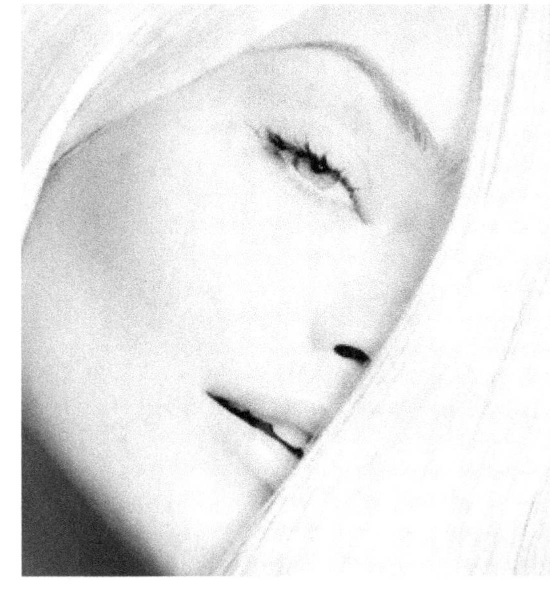

Your face is the first thing people look at. It will give a stranger their first impression of you and show others expression. Unfortunately, life shows up on your face. When you are tired, dehydrated, overexposed to sunlight, and show signs of stress it will be noticeable to others.

Eye Puffiness

Showing up to important events in life with a swollen face could dissipate your natural beauty and confidence. If my eyes are puffy in the morning there are several beauty industry tricks makeup artists pull out in an emergency.

Reducing puffiness:

1. One trick of the trade is aloe vera under the eyes. Not only does aloe aid in reducing puffiness, it can help with dark circles as well. Aloe firms the skin temporarily making it a soothing quick fix.

2. A cold washcloth or spoon can help reduce puffiness by increasing circulation.

3. Cool cucumbers and green tea bags both have anti-inflammatory properties. Lie down and relax with either on each eye, making sure both have been refrigerated and are nice and cool.

4. Hemorrhoid creams, such as Preparation H contain phenylephrine which will constrict blood vessels and reduce swelling. Try dabbing a little under each eye.

Dark Circles

Vitamin K used as a topical gel has been known to reduce dark circles under the eyes. Needed by the body for blood clotting and other important processes, this essential vitamin will reduce bruising, swelling, and those blasted dark circles under our eyes. However, if you DO have dark circles you shouldn't rely solely on creams and makeup, dark shading could be a sign your body is telling you it needs more sleep and/or better nutrition.

Exfoliate

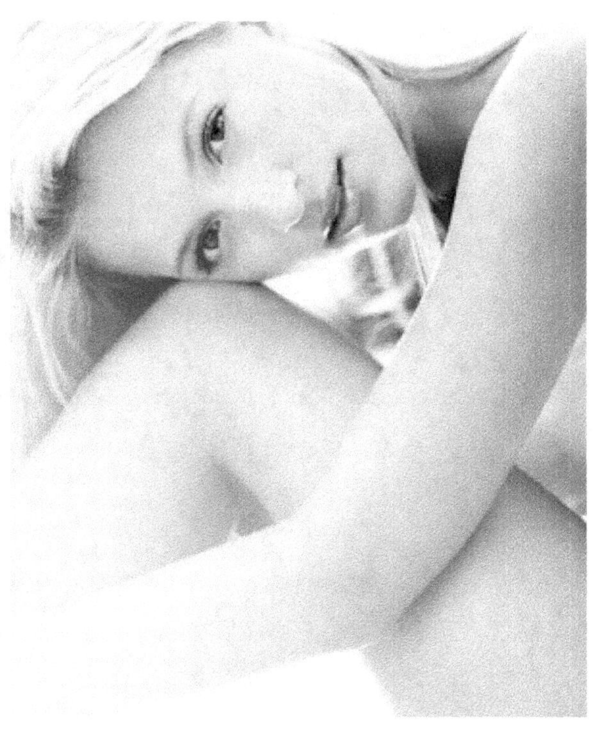

Exfoliating is an important method for maintaining radiating skin. Dead skin could cause a dull, ashy and lifeless appearance.

To remove dead skin, make wrinkles less visible, create a glowing complexion, rid toxins, and rejuvenate skin cells exfoliate the face and body often. Use a daily cleanser with micro exfoliating beads/grains to gently wash away dirt and makeup. Twice a week use a wash cloth or facial exfoliating pads to do more of the heavy lifting. Scrub in small circles, paying extra attention to the areas where wrinkles are most likely to occur such as crows feet and laugh lines. Exfoliating not only allows your skin to breathe easier but allows makeup to be applied smoothly.

Blemishes and Exfoliating

Have you ever had a pimple you've picked incessantly, leaving it irritated making it impossible for concealer to hide? It's imperative to exfoliate any blemish which decides to show, leaving the skin around the problem area smooth. Makeup can change the color of anything on skin including tattoos, but it can be difficult to change texture.

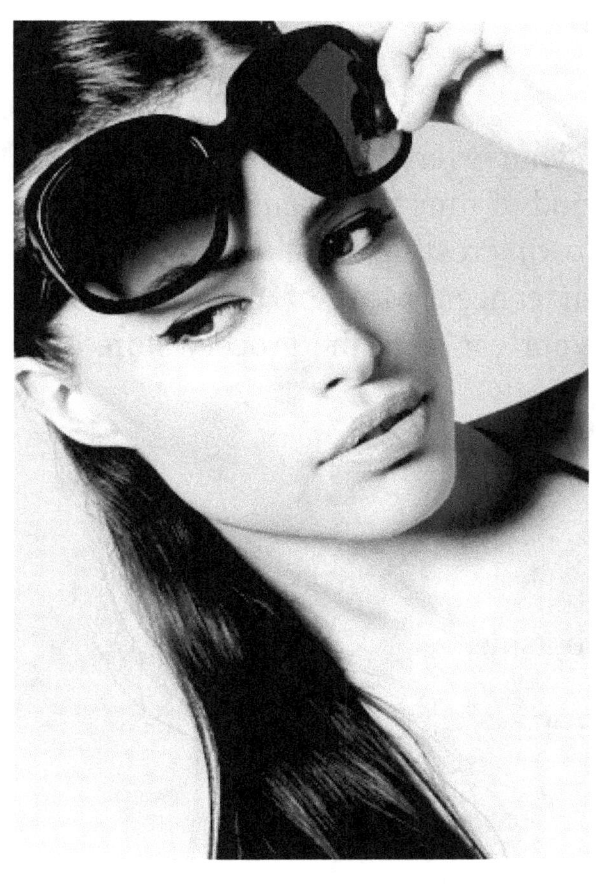

Sunglasses

Any exposure to sunlight, whether in your car, at the beach, and even in winter can cause your eyes to squint. Wearing sunglasses drastically reduces this reaction. You naturally wrinkle your eyes for protection when it's bright outside to shield yourself from harmful UV light, which can not only damage your eyes, but the thin layer of skin around your eyes. This extra damage and the act of squinting can cause fine lines and crows feet. Always cover your peepers!

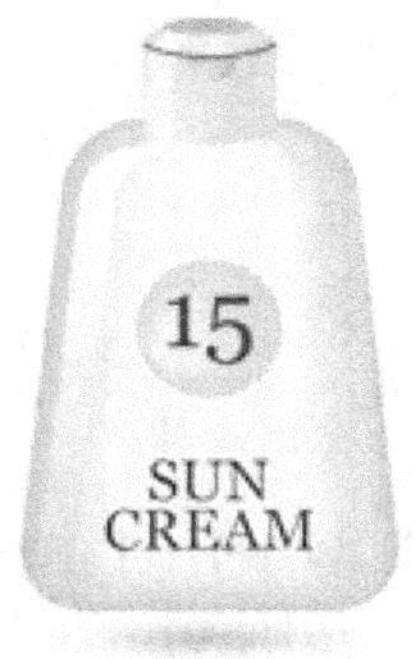

Sunscreen is necessary in your everyday beauty routine. UV rays over a prolonged period of time will damage fibers in the skin causing elastin break down creating wrinkles, aging, sun-spots, discoloration, and even cancer. Most of us don't realize driving and even walking to your car from the grocery store on a cloudy day can leave you exposed.

Wear sunscreen everyday.

Apply at least 15-20 minutes before you go outside.

Wear sunscreen with minimum of 30 to 50 SPF.

Don't forget arms, chest, ears and neck.

If you are outside for a prolonged period of time, grab the highest SPF sunscreen and reapply every two hours.

Make sunscreen a part of your beauty routine – SPF in lotions and face moisturizers.

Carry chap stick with SPF in it.

Clean your face with a gentle cleanser when you get back from sun exposure and use Aloe and Vitamin E.

Always have a doctor look at weird shaped and transforming moles, freckles, and dark spots.

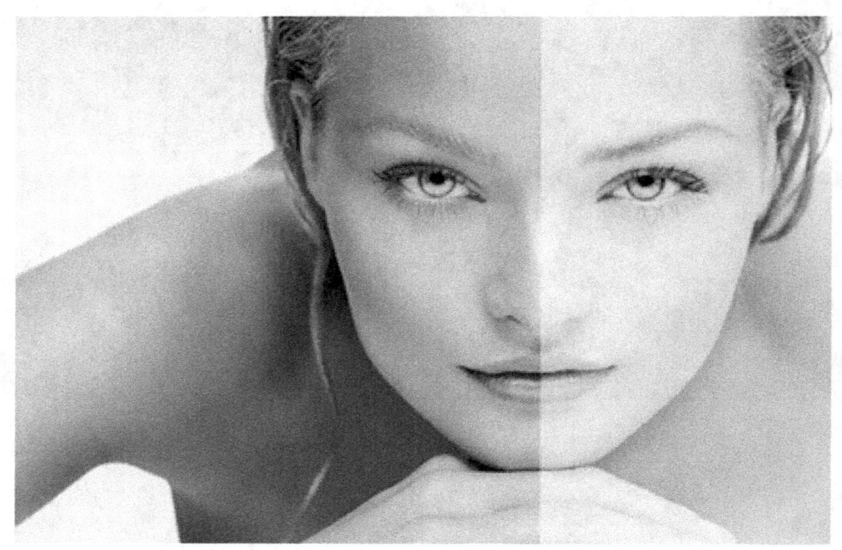

Bronzers

Bronzers can give you the look of a healthy tan without the sun while accenting your muscle tone. Applying to exposed skin leaves a beautiful, shimmery glow.

With a powder bronzer use a big powder brush for stroking chest, arms, and neck. Be careful not to over do it as too much powder can leave the skin looking fake or dirty. Adding a few extra vertical strokes in the middle of your bust can be appealing due to extra contouring. The same can be said for adding a little extra to your cheekbones for a bit more definition.

Bronzers also come in lotion form. This type is best applied straight out of the shower, allowing time to dry before getting dressed.

Pimples, Eww!

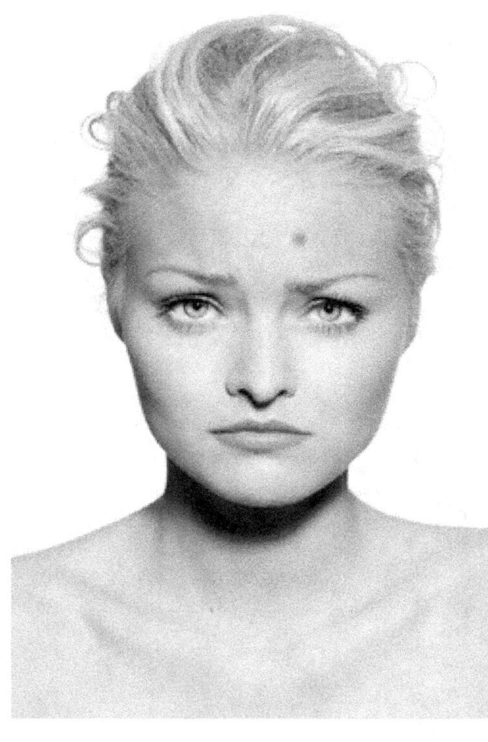

Pimples are a nightmare, not only for models but everyone. Seeming to show up at the most inopportune moments in life, the stress surrounding important events are one way to get the cheeky little devils. Other causes of acne: dirt, clogged pores, pressure (like helmets or sports bras), cosmetics, medication, hormones, and heredity. Fast food and pizza isn't necessarily good for your health, however, contrary to what most people believe it still hasn't been proven food is the cause of acne.

When a pimple begins to show, try to leave it alone. The more you touch it the more you irritate it. Dabbing benzoyl peroxide directly on the problem then leaving on over night will reduce swelling and dry the pimple out.

Plan your attack when puss has come to the surface. Clean the area with rubbing alcohol and use the tip of a cauterized needle or a skin care extractor to gently push the puss out. Always wash around the area as well as your hands after this process to prevent further breakouts. Then apply a benzoyl peroxide or salicylic acid topical cream leaving it over night. Exfoliating the around the area will be the finishing touch in the morning. The once horrid pimple should now be small, clean, and smooth - ready for makeup to cover any redness which may still be left.

Myths & Truths About Benzoyl Peroxide, Tea Tree Oil, and Toothpaste as Acne Remedies Benzoyl Peroxide Most popular, successful, and frequently used acne treatment – used in most acne medications as the active ingredient.

2 Generally inexpensive.

3 How it works: Benzoyl peroxide introduces oxygen into the pore which will kill the bacteria population.

4 It also rids the follicle of excess dead skin cells – therefore preventative.

5 Must be used continuously.

6 Most common side effects are dryness and flaking.

1 **Tea Tree Oil** Can kill bacteria and has fewer side effects then benzoyl peroxide.

2 Takes longer than benzoyl peroxide to show improvement.

3 Has to be diluted to less than 5%. Undiluted tea tree oil can cause skin irritation, redness, blistering, over drying, and itching.

4 The research of using tea tree oil has not been as conclusive as benzoyl peroxide.

1 **Toothpaste** The common myth of toothpaste being used is most likely due to its triclosan contact, which effectively kills bacteria. However, the other ingredients can do more harm than good.

2 Toothpaste can make your pimple look worse, often leaving it sore, inflamed, and red the next day.

Salt Scrubs

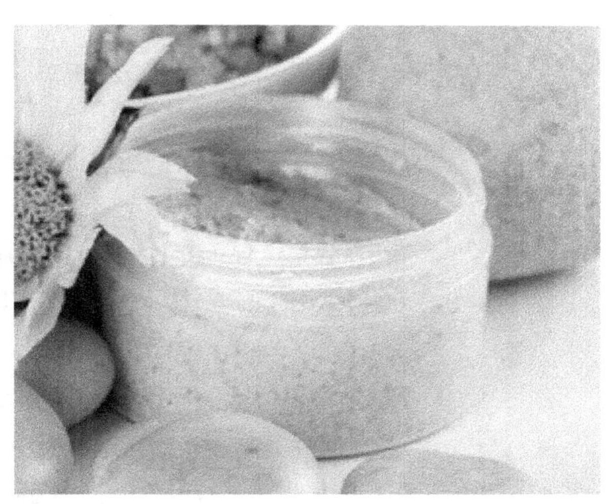

If you haven't tried salt scrubs you maybe missing out on the most luxurious your skin can feel. I'm always at my sexiest, softest, and most radiant after using a scented scrub.

Salt scrubs act as a skin buffer to remove dead, dull skin which in turn reveals your younger, more youthful skin underneath. It also cleans pours better then soaps or cleansers, allowing skin to breath easier. Salt scrubs stimulate blood circulation, helping future skin regenerate while removing daily toxins and strengthening skin tissue.

There are many different types of salt scrubs. The best and my personal favorite is dead sea salt because it's less refined, leaving more natural minerals to be absorbed. These minerals include magnesium, potassium, bromine, calcium chloride and sodium, all vital to youthful and healthy looking skin.

Salt scrubs can be expensive, however, there is a solution -- you can make your own at home. By making your own you have the freedom to add essential oils of your choice, such as lavender or vanilla, as well as it can make a great gift for friends and family. It's as easy as filling a clean jar with your choice of salt and an oil which is good for your skin. Oils good for your skin include; almond oil, coconut oil, grape seed oil, safflower oil, jojoba oil, avocado oil, peanut oil, rose hip oil, sesame oil, macadamia nut oil, sunflower oil or olive oil. All that remains is filling the rest of the jar with a few drops of your favorite essential oil for scent.

Cocoa Butter

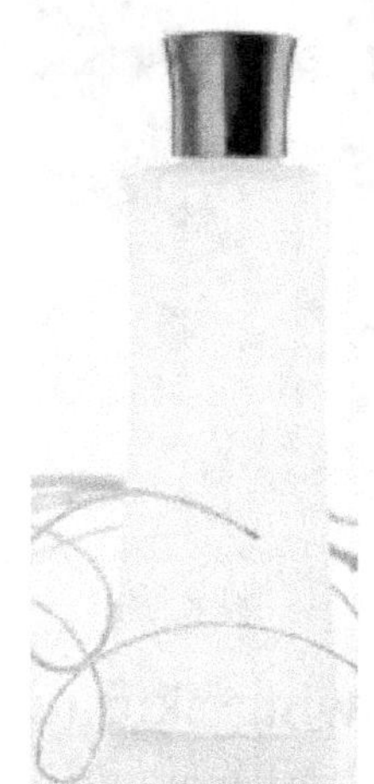

Cocoa butter lotion is a great choice to have as a body moisturizer. Naturally containing tons of vitamins like A, C and E, as well as phytochemicals working as mega antioxidants, which are all beneficial to skin's health. The fat in cocoa butter acts as a natural emollient, giving suppleness to skin lipids (aids in stretch mark prevention) and acting as a barrier to protect skin from the harsh elements the environment can throw at you. Chocolate (cocoa) in general should be in your beauty diet because it contains polyphenols and other compounds which possess antioxidant properties ridding the body of free radicals -- toxins which come from pollution, smoking, stress, and sun damage.

Since cocoa butter has been proven to be mild it can be used on most skin types. Even companies like Johnson & Johnson trust its use in their baby products. Doctors also recommend it for treatment of skin ailments like eczema and dermatitis.

"I Don't Sweat, I Glow"

Women hate to sweat. Melting makeup, embarrassing stains, and smelling are the antithesis of femininity. However, no matter how inconvenient, sweat is wonderful for your skin and health. Benefits such as reducing muscle stiffness, burning extra calories, increasing blood circulation, promoting relaxation/well-being, and improving your immune system come with sweating. To give skin a kick, go for a 15 minute sweat session a few times a week.

There are different options for increasing sweat other than exercise such as a steam room or sauna. I prefer a steam room over the sauna because I find it easier to handle and I love the moisture. Steam rooms are also good for your respiratory system. However, people with breathing problems should probably opt for the sauna instead. Still, consult your doctor before using either.

After stepping into a steam room or sauna, you will immediately start to sweat to maintain your basal body temperature of 98.6 F. At first your body is able to fend off the heat but eventually it can no longer dissipate the heat and your body temperature inevitability begins to rise. Blood is then more forcefully shunted toward the surface of your skin causing a heavier sweat which can rinse out your pours. The increased blood circulation also brings more oxygen and nutrients to your skin's surface.

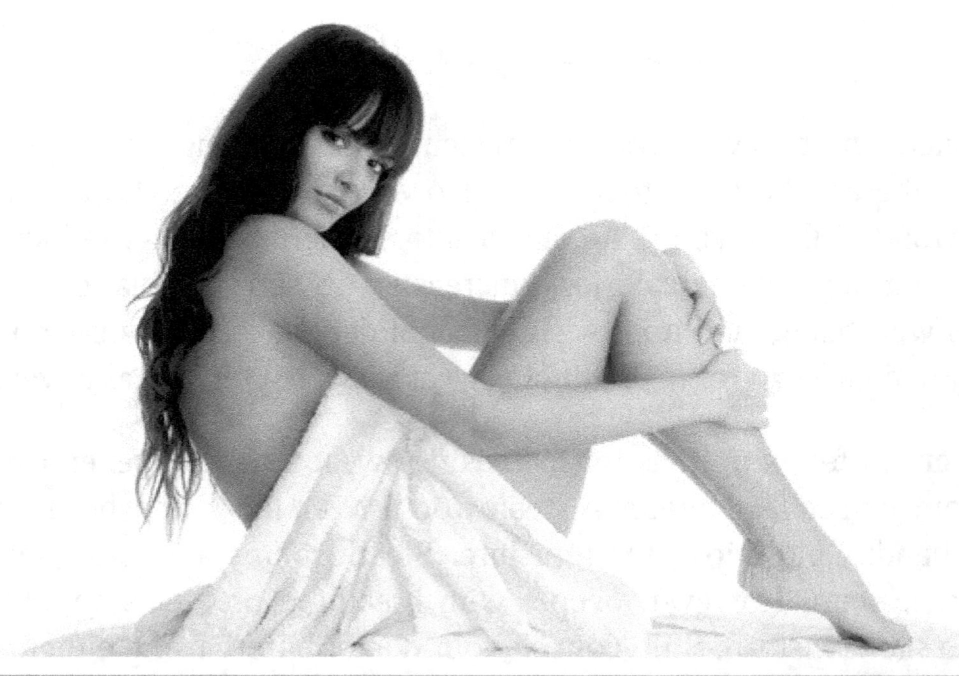

Pat Dry Don't Rub

To help retain natural moisture after bathing, pat dry then apply a moisturizer within three minutes of getting out of the shower. Gently blotting the skin helps lock in and retain moisture and is less irritating to dry sensitive skin. This insures sexy, soft, and touchable skin.

Dry Flaky Lips

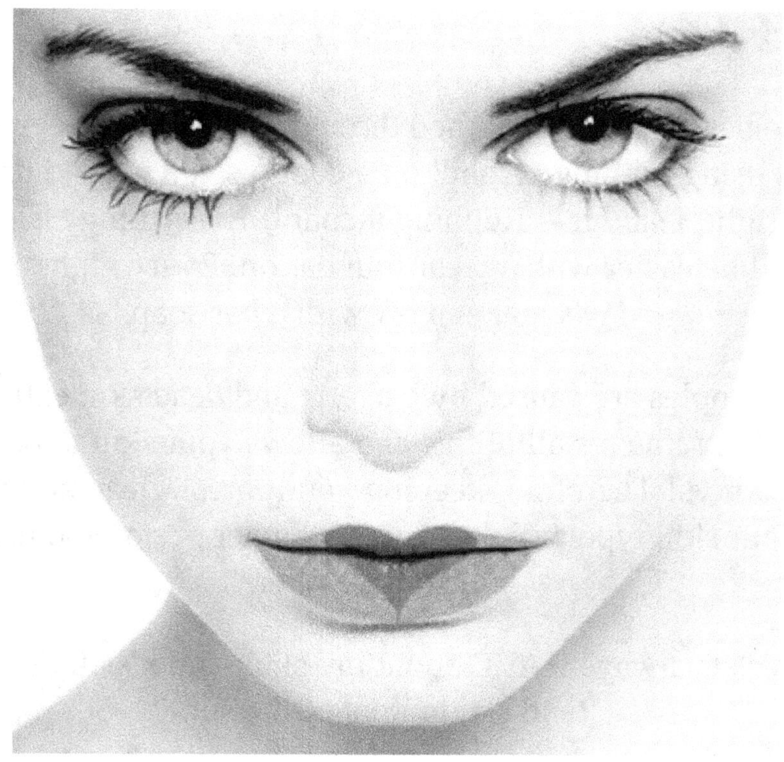

Dry cracked lips are usually a sign of dehydration and could also be caused by harsh weather. No picture can be pretty with a cracked pucker. The way to treat needy lips is to coat them with petroleum jelly, then leave it on for about 10 minutes to soften. Next use a warm damp washcloth to rub away the dead skin cells. Lastly, use another coat of lip balm on your kisser.

Muah!

Pro Tips

Piper Hinson - Model/Actress/Muscian

"One of the best tricks I've learned through the years to keep my skin looking gorgeous is using rubbing alcohol on a cotton swab instead of an expensive toner. That's right, I said it -- Rubbing alcohol! Everything else (I.E. putting on makeup) will be easier with a clear foundation. Every night, I also wash my day's makeup off with a bar soap."

"Acne and pimples are caused by bacteria and dead skin cells clogging pores. Rubbing alcohol removes all of this and allows your skin to be totally dry and free of any germys! Therefore, keeping your pores "clean and clear and under control!" Your skin type will determine whether or not you need to put on a moisturizer after."

"Makeup artists always RAVE about my skin, and it's all due to this practice! (and staying out of the sun)"

Alex Noiret - Model

"For glowing, clear skin, I wash my face at least three times a day with ice cold water. Occasionally, I will use some Neutrogena "heat glow," a soft soft scrub which I'm able to use hot water with. This opens the pores to allow the chemicals to work, but I ALWAYS splash/rinse with ice cold water. I also always wear sunscreen and watch what I eat by staying away from greasy foods for clear healthy skin."

Lisa Lakatos - Model/Actress
Former Deal or No Deal case model

"Protect your eyes! Sunglasses and eye cream with SPF are key when it comes to avoiding sun damage. Signs of aging are most noticeable in the eye area. Many young women don't include eye cream in their beauty regime...yet, moisturizing the eyes is just as important as the face. I use a hydrating eye cream every night before bed and one with SPF every morning before I leave the house."

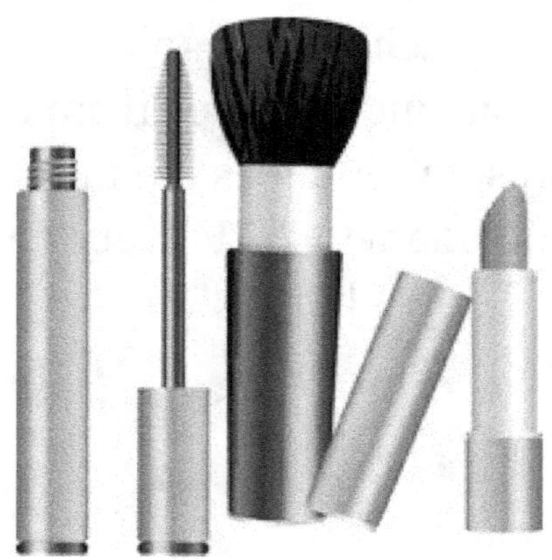

Chapter Two: MAKEUP

Makeup is used to accent your best features, hide blemishes, and make a Plain Jane into a diva. Like a designer, you can use makeup for transitioning an everyday appearance into a pretty piece of décor. When you want to look your best, creating perfect skin and highlighting your favorite features are important techniques to harness for all of life's occasions.

If You Don't Have Time Makeup

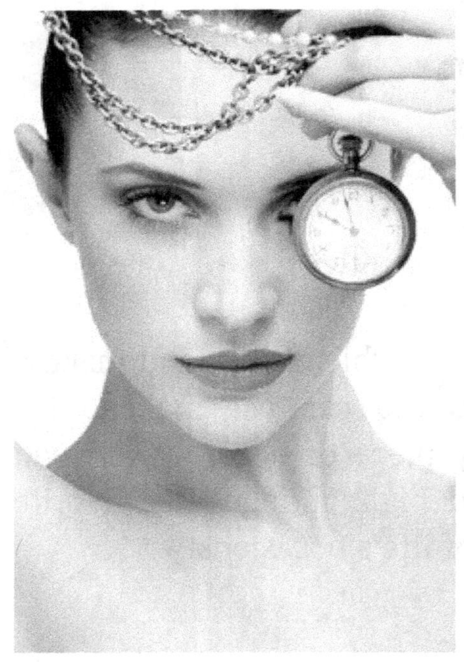

Don't have time to apply full makeup? Here are a few quick tricks to maintain a fresh, glowing look in a hurry.

stayfresh

What to do:

Moisturize: Grab your face lotion and your foundation. Squeeze a small amount of both into your palm. Rub your hands together mixing the two. Apply by rubbing evenly to your face (like you would with sunblock). This will even out your skin tone.

Blush: The essential to making your quick makeup job a success. Blush is used to give you a healthier look, and to help define your facial structure. This will also brighten and accentuate your most prominent features.

Lip Gloss: It's always good to keep emergency lip gloss in your purse.

Mascara: A quick coat of mascara will complete your look by making your eyes pop.

Contouring

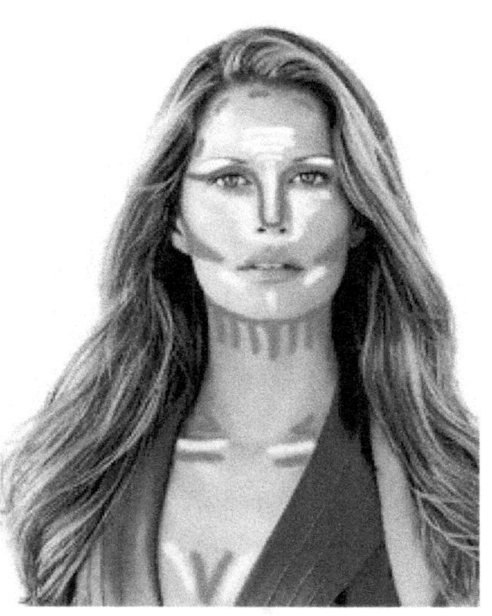

Makeup artists have many tricks to help achieve your ultimate level of beauty. They also have secrets to help improve in the areas you lack. If you don't have a chiseled jaw line or cheek bones, there are ways of using makeup to help your features look more defined than they really are. Like an artist who uses paints and color pencils, you can use shading to achieve this.

What To Do You will need a powder or bronzer which is a few shades darker then your skin tone. Start by applying your normal base. Cover up blemishes to even your skin tone. Then, using a blush brush, apply the darker shade powder as you would a blush, but instead of on your cheeks, apply to the concave below your cheekbone. Fill in from your ear lobe to about halfway down the cheekbone. Next, apply the bronzing powder under and along your jawline and neck for a more sexy, chiseled look. Go over it a few times but not heavily -- don't give away your trick. When you have achieved the proper shading, blush can be applied on the apples of your cheekbones. Depending on your facial structure, the bronzer and blush may over lap.

Giving Your Eyes Extra Pop

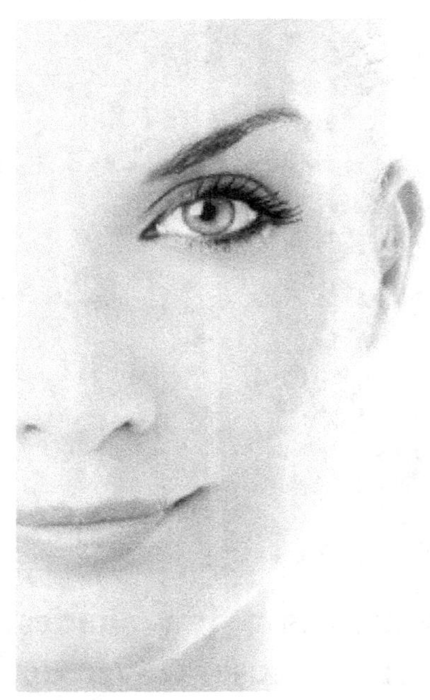

Because everyday is different, there is not a standard way to do makeup. Depending on the occasion or how your feeling will determine the day's strategy. You could be tired, in a certain mood, swinging by the grocery store or out on the town. That said, having your eyes pop adds intensity which can be ravishing to your admirers whatever the circumstance.

If your tired use a light pearl/white/pastel color eye shadow in the inside corners of your eyes. This will make the eyes look fresh and more open.

When you want to wear sexier makeup, use eyeliner by lining the inside bottom lid with a black or brown. This makes the eyes stand out to draw people in. This method works best in two coats.

For eye brightening, line the inside lid near the bottom lash line with a shimmery white eyeliner to open up the eye. This technique works well for women who have smaller eyes to create the illusion of larger ones.

Having a clean, plucked eyebrow will help make your eyes stand out and make your overall appearance look more put together. There is no substitute for natural eyebrows.

The reason we want to spend extra time on our eyes is because it's the first thing people view. Eyes show expression and let people know how you are feeling, your thoughts, and your intentions. We want to make our eyes pop to show we are healthy, happy, and fresh.

Don't be afraid to have a little color on the apples of the cheekbones (petal pink). It really brightens up your face. Adding a little color gives you the just-back-from-the-beach-look boost.

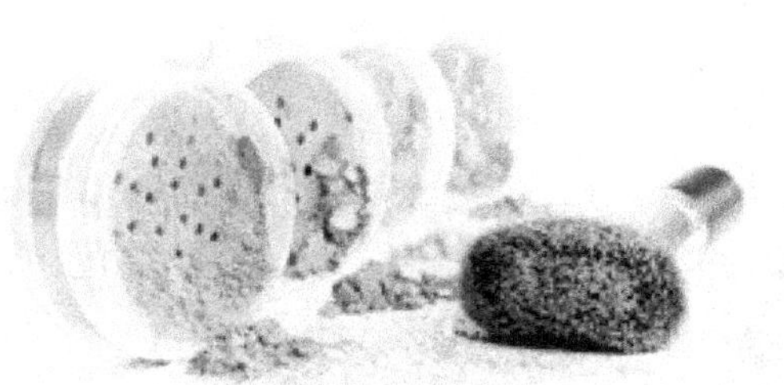

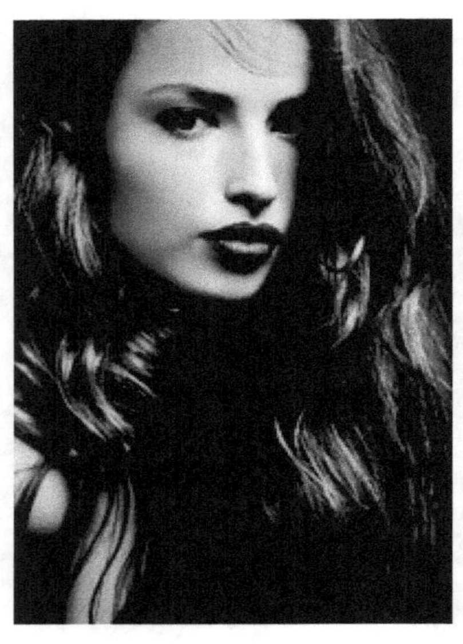

Darker Eyes or Darker Lips

Makeup can take years to master since there are many effects. Unfortunately, it's counterproductive to wear all the techniques at the same time. For example, having a very dark, smokey eye, a very dark lipstick might give the look of "wearing too much." Makeup is here to enhance features. No need to overcompensate. Pulling out all the tricks of the eyes and the lips could make our admirers notice the makeup which, potentially, will undo all our hard work. We wouldn't want to take the focus off our natural beauty and best features.

What To Do
I recommend to do one or the other. Choose to have a darker eye with a lighter lip (lighter lip gloss) or a lighter eye (light/pastels or earthy eye shadows and mascara) with a darker lip. Both options will showcase which feature you like most about yourself and both are incredibly sexy and feminine.

Eye Drops

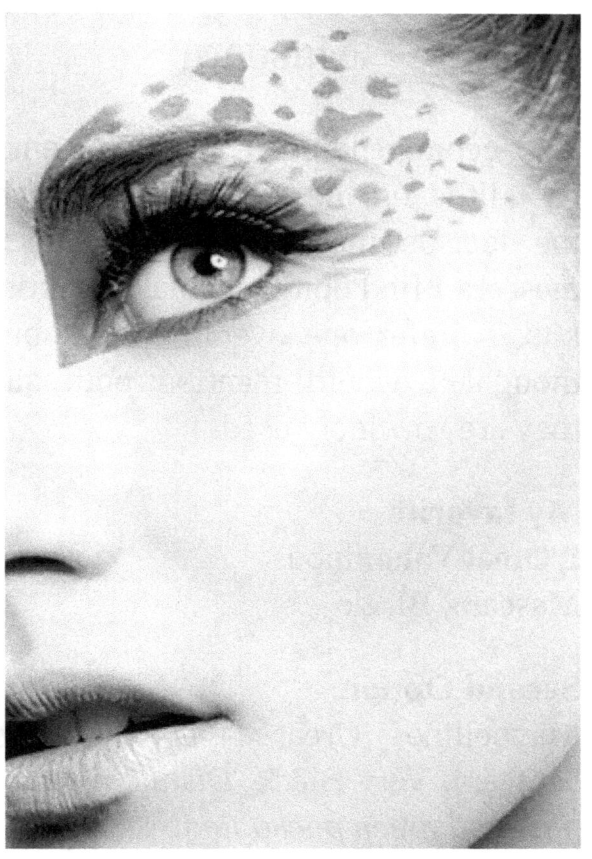

The first step for bright eyes is to use a few drops of an eye redness reducer. Products like Visine or Clear Eyes will do the trick. By taking away redness, you will appear to glow and look fresh. White eyes let people know you are healthy and well-rested. Remember to apply eye drops before adding makeup or moisturizer, taking away the potential of smudging or smearing a beautifully finished face.

Mascara

Recommending a product seems a little on the advertising side, but the fact is there are two brands of mascara I find dominate makeup artists' kits. I prefer one over the other but I thought I would mention both since they are so widely used.

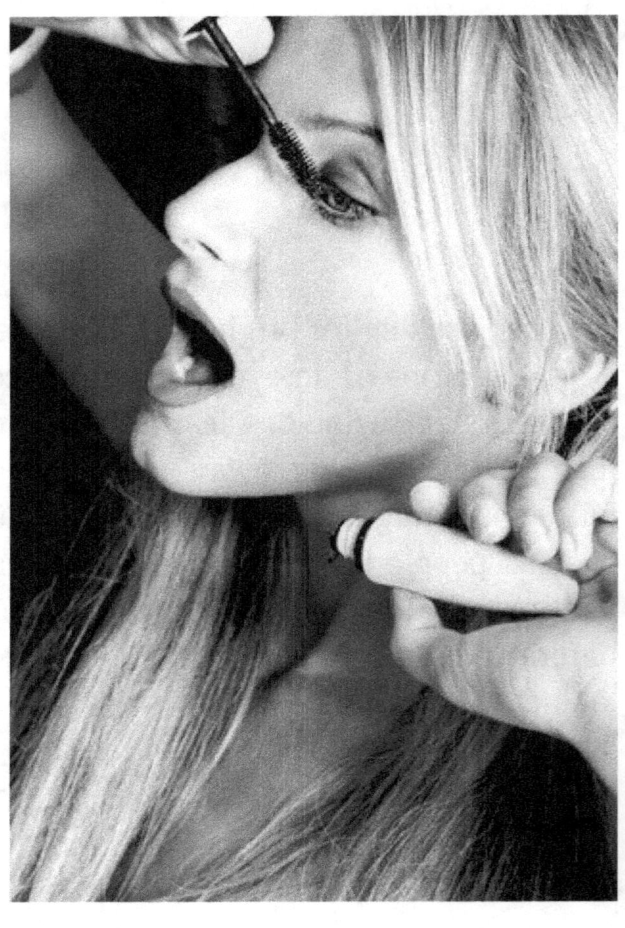

My favorite:
L'Oreal Voluminous
Mascara, Black

Second Option:
Maybelline Great Lash Washable Mascara, Very Black. *Distinctive bright pink and green packaging.*

These two products are so regarded because of two simple facts: they don't clump and go on thick. Using these in waterproof will create flirty lashes which won't run or smudge.

While holding the applicator, start at the base of your upper eyelashes. In a rotating motion, slightly move the applicator back and forth while slowly rotating the brush from the base to the ends. Let the first coat dry for one to two minutes. Then add another coat of mascara. Use an eyelash separator if the mascara is thicker in some places or if you have clumping.

Wet Your Makeup Sponge

When applying a base of foundation and concealer, wet the makeup sponge before application. This will make the foundation go on lighter, ensuring the foundation doesn't look too "cakey." You don't need to use a lot of water or soak the sponge. Run the sponge under the faucet quickly to dampen it. Then squeeze some of the excess water out. You can apply more foundation if needed. Some foundations are unnecessarily thick. Most girls don't realize you don't need a lot of foundation to balance out skin tones and cover blemishes. When covering a blemish it will look worse if you have three layers of concealer as opposed to a correct layer to began.

Eye Colors, Eye Shadows

Dark eyes look good in **grays**, **blues**, **purples**, and **greens**.

Light eyes look good in brown, **taupe**, and **bronze** shades.

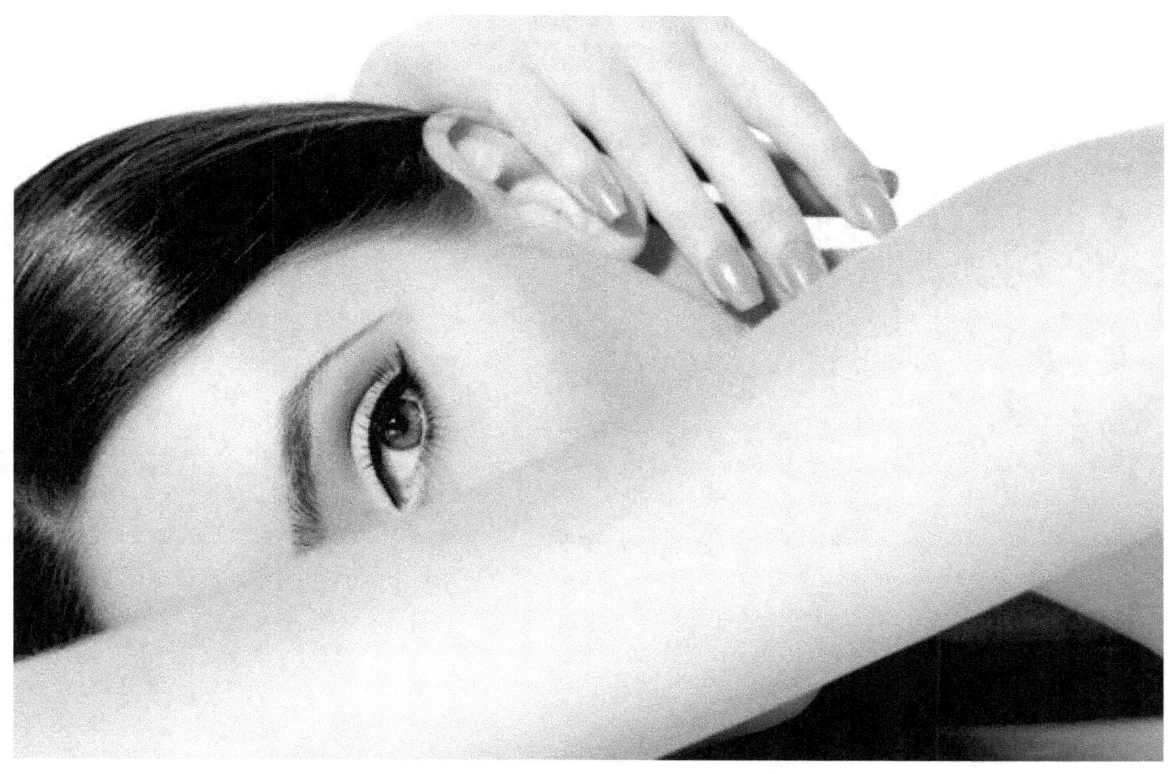

Eyebrows

Great eyebrows can make you look more glamorous by giving your face a lift without surgery. This is a natural beauty enhancer. The top three ways to get perfect brows are old fashioned plucking, waxing, and new-age threading. An ancient Eastern technique, threading has recently gained popularity in the West by using a pure cotton thread to roll over the hairline removing unwanted hair at follicle level.

If you want to mix it up when it comes to eyebrows, try plucking and sometimes threading. Waxing is a wonderful method to clean up the brow line but can be harsh on the delicate skin around the eyes. Threading is less harsh while it gets the hard-to-see tiny hairs creating a very straight line. However, there is always a risk to let someone else mess with your brows. Beware of having anyone get near your eyebrows without a lot experience. If they leave your eyebrows too thin, it's a nightmare to grow back.

I find most women haven't heard of eyebrow razors, let alone put one to practical use. Eyebrow razors are cheap, single razors usually with a plastic handle. You can buy them at any beauty supply store and they typically come in packages of four. They are fantastic for shaving off the small, almost invisible hairs near your temples and brow line in between beauty brow visits; a great finishing touch to your eyebrow routine.

Perfect Brows by Plucking

1 Have a clean face to work with. Use a small brush, like a mascara wand, to brush your brow hair upward and trim with small eyebrow scissors. Trimming only a small amount at time, until you have more practice. If you cut too much off it will leave you with bald spots.

2 Look closely at the shape. Your brow should begin at your tear duct, peak at the outer edge of your iris, and end at the outer corner of your eye. Hold a pencil in line with the outer side of your iris and note where the peak of your arch naturally occurs. From the arch to the outer corner of the eye, your brow should fall in a straight or slightly curved line, depending on the look you're trying to achieve.

3 Using your tweezers, pluck the hairs below the brow line and the obvious ones which don't belong above the brow line. Make sure you pluck along with the hair growth. When you start to pluck a shape, brush often and follow your natural line. Be careful when following brow trends, like really thick or thin brows, because trends always change. Do what looks the best to your face. Makeup artists have often told me to pluck one hair at a time. You never know

which one missing will change the whole shape. Don't forget when plucking one side, often look at the other side to make sure what you want to achieve can balance on both sides. The right and left side hair follicles aren't exact.

4 When finished plucking, use a toner over the brow or an astringent to kill any bacteria.

5 Lastly, fill in sparse areas with a brow filling technique of your choice. If using a freshly sharpened brow pencil, use light quick strokes to make your brow line appear fuller. Brow powder's will give thin brows overall definition and is great for a more natural look. If using a brow brush, sweep powder following the hair growth on each brow (my favorite technique). If you're a brow novice, a tinted brow gel is a foolproof way to keep brows in place. Lightly coat brows using upward and outward strokes. Wipe off any excess and allow it to set.

Applying a Base

Foundations and Concealers

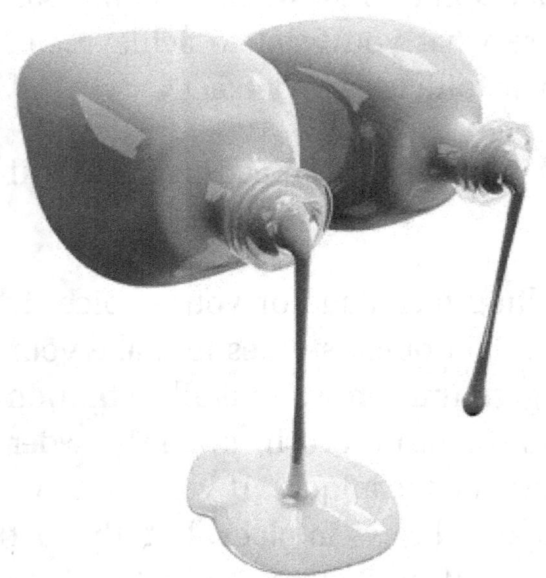

A beautiful base is meant to even skin tone, give glowing healthy looking skin, and act as a primer. Think of your face as a blank easel and your makeup as your paint. After all, they don't call them makeup "artists" for nothing.

Choosing Foundation

To avoid looking orange or ashy, you need to choose a foundation which matches your skin tone perfectly. Foundations will either have undertones of pink or yellow. If your undertones are somewhere in the middle you may have to blend two foundations to get the perfect match. This technique is completely acceptable and encouraged. Most beauty counters will be able to give you exactly what you need.

To match foundation to your skin, test it on your neck and chest. The chest is ultimately where the foundation will have to meet and blend, making it the optimal testing place, instead of your hand which, may have a different tone.

1 Start with a clean face and moisturize. Use a moisturizer which works with your skin combination (oily, dry, normal). Make sure it has an SPF over 15 in it. Sun damage can occur during any season and any situation, even if exposed for a few minutes.

2 Apply your foundation with a damp makeup sponge or foundation brush evenly. Use the clean side of the makeup sponge to blend into your hairline, around your jawline, and into your neck. If you don't blend into surrounding areas of the face, you could end up with an unwanted "mask" look.

3 Dab concealer under your eyes and on any blemish or discolored areas either with your finger or a concealer brush. Use your makeup sponge again to lightly go over the blemished areas to blend the two shades together.

4 To eliminate shine and set your base, use a loose powder by applying with a powder brush. It works best if you dip your brush into the powder and give it a shake/tap to knock some of the extra powder out.

5 Contouring your face is optional but as a last step you can grab a bronzer or a darker powder and brush a few strokes just under cheek bones, top of hairline, and jawline lightly.

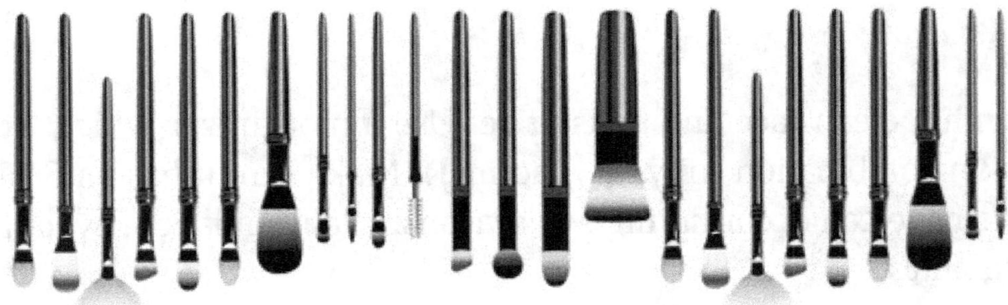

Makeup Brushes

On every set, makeup artists come armed with cosmetic tools and brushes. Makeup brushes are essential to applying makeup as well as helping with precision, blending, and accuracy. Always use good quality makeup brushes and avoid grabbing any old thing lying in the drawer. Investing in good brushes will not only change the way makeup can look on you, but a higher grade brush can last up to ten years, if taken care of properly.

There are different types of brushes for different makeup applications, as well as different hair bristle types and levels of quality. The best quality brushes use natural hair because the bristles are soft and can absorb makeup. This is ideal for blushes, eye shadows, and powders. Synthetic hair is non-absorbent which can be suitable for foundations and concealers.

Foundation Brush

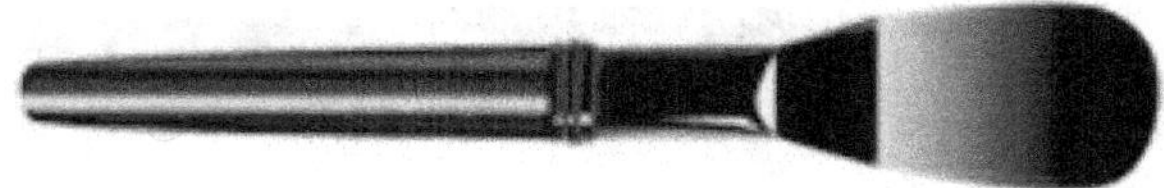

Foundation brushes are usually flat-shaped and made from synthetic materials. Great for applying foundation to give an even, flawless look. Your application will go on thicker with a brush than with a sponge making it perfect for a night out or camera ready.

Concealer Brush

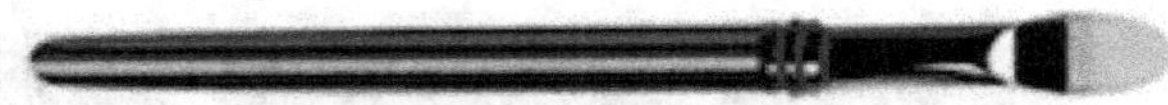

This brush has a flat and tapered shape with a synthetic bristle. It is perfect for applying concealer under-the-eyes, cleaning up under-the-eye after you have applied dark eye shadows, covering blemishes, and applying cream based eye shadows.

Powder Brush

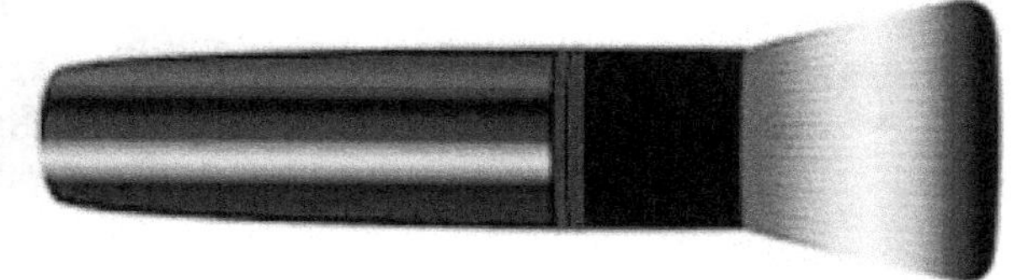

These are the biggest of the brushes. The powder brush is fat, round, and made from natural hair. Powder brushes are used for applying loose powder to eliminate shine. Not only used for getting rid of shine it can also be used to apply bronzers and body makeup because of it's surface area.

Blush Brush

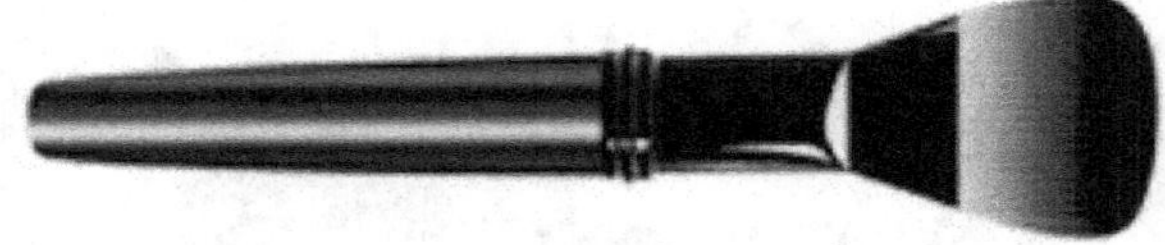

Similar to the powder brush, the blush brush is smaller and curves more like a dome. Made from natural hair and the dome shape perfect for contouring. This is an essential brush to have in your makeup tool kit, as blush gives your face a healthier look. I also use a blush brush after applying eye shadow, to go over my eyes with it as a final blending technique.

Eye Shadow Brush

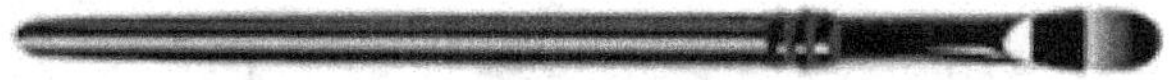

There are multiple shapes and types of eye shadow brushes but they should always have natural hair bristles. Makeup artists use a medium to large-sized eye shadow brush for highlighting (under the brow or the inner corners of the eye), as well as blending. A small/medium bullet-shaped brush can be used for the contours of the eye, and general eyeshadow application.

Eyebrow Brush

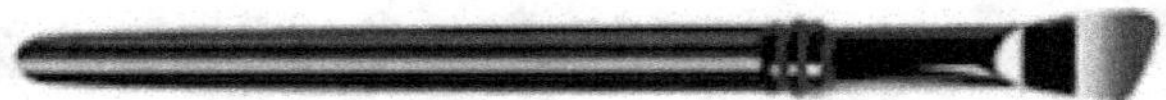

This brush is the most firm of all the brushes and is flat and cut at an angle. Using this brush instead of an eyebrow liner can create a more natural looking brow. Dab the brush into an earthy color brown, close to your eyebrow shade, going over each brow a couple of times to build an even line.

Eye Liner Brush

These are soft, fine, natural haired brushes which are thin, long, and come to a point. Nothing compares to using this brush when applying liquid or cream eye liner.

Smudge Brush

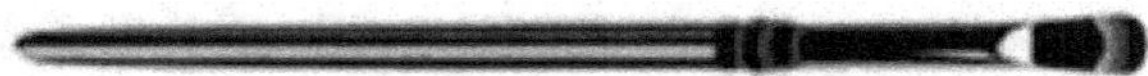

These brushes can be made of foam with a pointed dome shape or a short natural haired bristle. Use it to smudge eyeliner, contour dark eye shadows, and to soften any hard lines.

Lip Brush

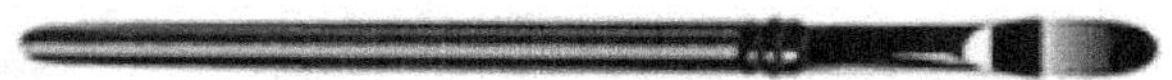

These brushes are usually thin, flat and synthetic like a concealer brush. Although you can use lipstick from the package or case, using a lip brush can give you excellent precision. Perfect for applying dark and very red lipsticks as messing up with these colors will be noticeable.

Fan Brush

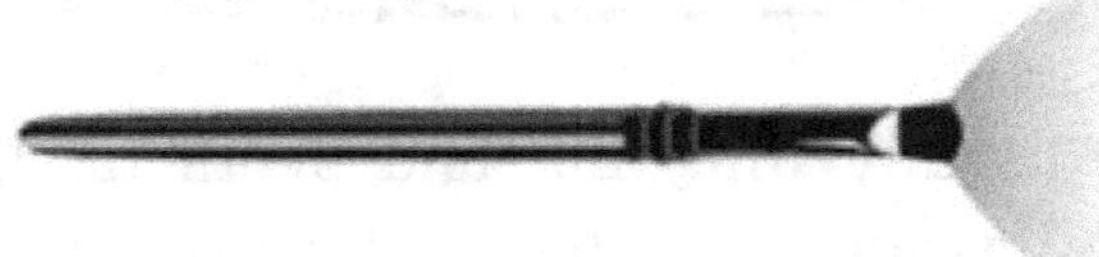

These are shaped like a fan and made from natural hair. The fan brush can be used to dust away excess makeup or apply darker powders and bronzers. They are great for blushes too.

> You only have to replace better quality brushes once about every 10 years, if taken care of properly.

Although, all these brushes are amazing to have in your makeup bag, it can get costly to buy them all at once. If you are just starting your makeup brush collection I recommend these few essentials to get you started:

1. Concealer Brush
2. Blush Brush
3. Eye Shadow Medium Brush
4. Smudge Brush
5. Powder Brush

Try looking around online to price compare but avoid cheap drug store brushes which you will have to be replace weekly and hinder you from creating the proper effect.

How To Clean Brushes

Cleaning makeup brushes is as important as washing your hands. Brushes are harbingers for germs, bacteria, dirt, and grime, which in turn can make you sick, give you infections, and cause breakouts.

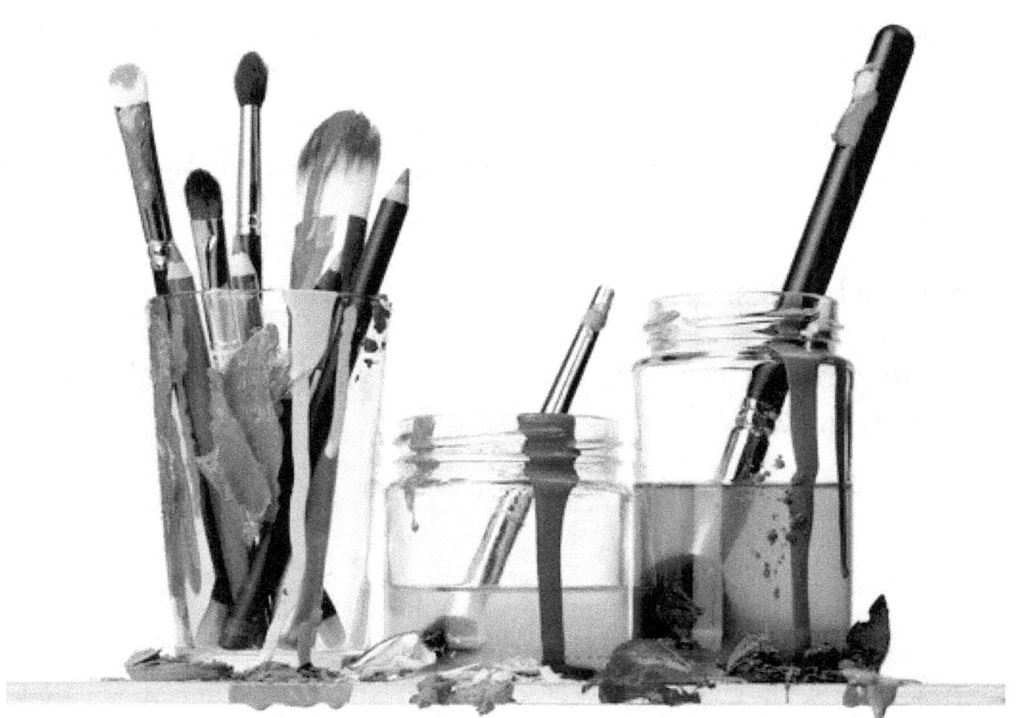

Clean makeup brushes about once every two weeks using either shampoo or a brush cleanser. Make sure not to use bar or hand soaps which will strip the brushes.

1 Wet the brush and dip it into a small bowl with the brush cleanser or shampoo and warm water. Use 1 ½ cups of water to one teaspoon of shampoo.

2 Rinse the brush under the faucet until thoroughly clean. Then squeeze and towel dry.

3 Reshape the bristles.

4 Lay flat to air dry. Do not stand the brushes up to dry, as this will cause mold and bacteria growth.

Apply Makeup In Natural Light

Since dim or florescent light can change how makeup looks, makeup artists set up their stations in an area with the best lighting. Bad light can make it difficult to see if makeup has gone on evenly and has the potential for a heavy application. If your makeup looks good in natural light, it will look good in most situations. Find a big window to set up shop near. If sitting near a window isn't an option, go outside with a mirror for your final touches after applying makeup.

Celebrity Teeth

Having a perfect bright smile enhances attractiveness. Which is why celebs and models pay top dollar to get their teeth pearly white. The first time I whitened my teeth, I couldn't believe what was staring back at me. The confidence of a bright smile which is uninhibited adds volumes to self-esteem. It changed my life.

> Try using a desensitizing toothpaste like Sensodyne after a whitening treatment to help with uncomfortable tooth sensitivity.

There are different options to a bright, white smile:

You can make an appointment with your dentist and do an office laser treatment. This is usually the most expensive way to go but immediately effective and can last the longest out of any of the whitening options.

1 This method leaves your teeth the most sensitive.

2 Another option is the use of bleaching trays. Your dentist can make a mold of your teeth to make the tray comfortable and effective. You can also find generic trays at your local drug store. Leave the tray in your mouth over night usually taking three to four days to see results.

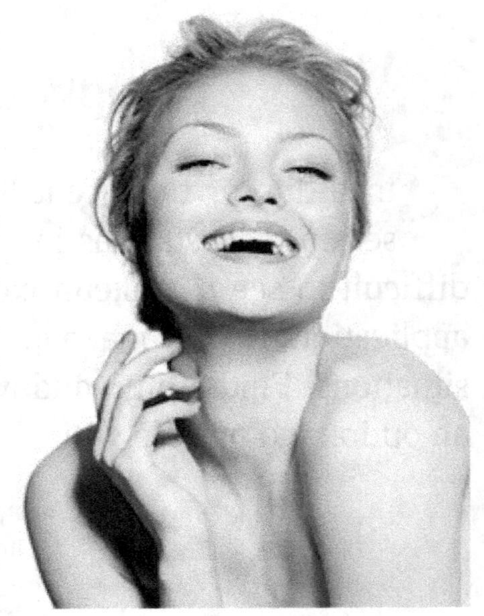

3 My preferred method is whitening strips. This method also happens to be the cheapest (around $20-40 for a package). There are more options for teeth whitening and home remedies like hydrogen peroxide and baking soda, however, whitening strips is what works for me. You can see results in about a week the first time using this product. For touch ups, you can in results in a few sessions. They feel non-evasive as you only have to put a strip on for a half hour. You can also drink water, put on makeup, and live life while they are in your mouth, unlike other methods, leaving you with a bright, confident smile.

Pro Tips

Wendi San George - Celebrity Hairstylist/Makeup Artist

"As the past makeup/hair designer for NBC's Deal or No Deal and many other current primetime shows, I have one trick that I don't leave home with out - Ardell lashes!! I use them with black duo adhesive so it dries into a instant eye liner. Which is an amazing instant fast framing of one's eye. I never leave home with out them myself and I would never send a client in front of the camera with out wearing a pair... or two. Yes, that's right! You can double them up for drama. It's an amazing tool."

Ashly Walsh - Model/Actress

Smokey eye tip (my favorite tip from an amazing makeup artist, Kim Bragalone):

"Try lining the top of your lids with a light gold hued eyeshadow to brighten. Next, fill in the lower lids with a cream pinkish eye shadow. Then line the bottom of your lids with a heavy line of a dark eye pencil. After, try taking a small makeup brush to blend up to the eye crease and you will have a nice light smokey eye. Always remember to use a lash curler and mascara. I also love to use a mascara primer first, it will add thickness and depth to mascara. Smashbox makes a great one. It's worth it!"

Kristina Nicole Anderson - Hairstylist/Makeup Artist

"There are three steps I recommend to do before makeup application: exfoliate, use a toner, and apply a SPF moisturizer. These step will ensure an even makeup application. I also make sure I have a base before I apply eyeshadows."

"When on television or on a photo shoot make sure to always know which areas to highlight and which areas to shade. Highlight areas you want standing out! It's important to highlight the areas according to your facial shape and structure."

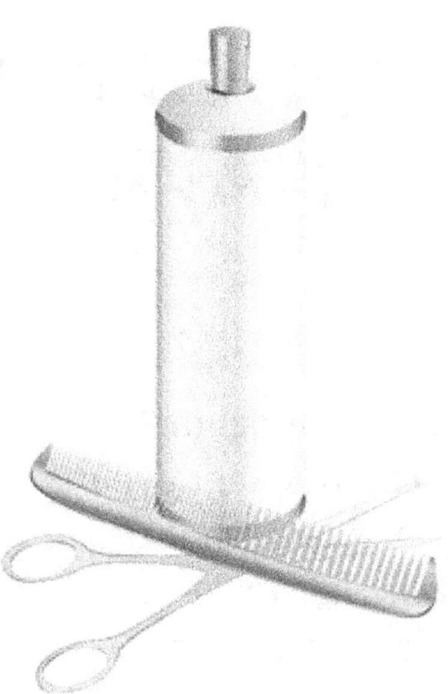

Chapter Three: HAIR

Part of a complete beauty routine includes hair maintenance. Hair care, styling, and products are all integral parts of a personalized look. The smallest change to a boring braid or predictable curl can give an air of trend setting style and sophistication. Hair makes it's own statement. Try these helpful tips for healthy, stylish, and glamorous hair.

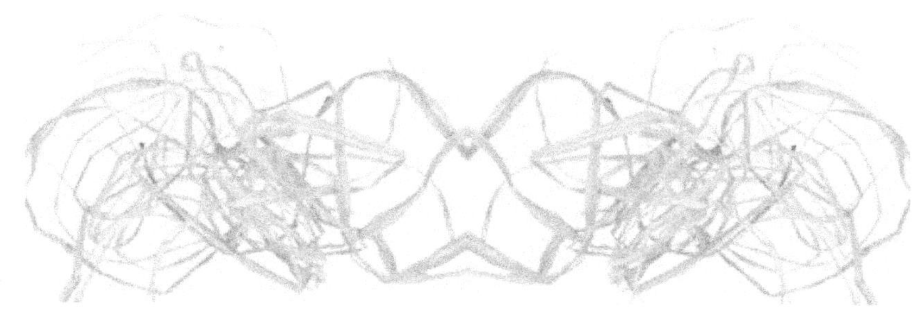

Dry Hair Rescue

Daily Life can take it's toll on hair. Hair gets flat-ironed, curled, pulled on, and blown-out, with sometimes no break, as your routine can be everyday. When you notice your hair is starting to feel like straw, it's time to put on a deep conditioner or hair mask overnight. There are many products out there to fit all budgets. If you're strapped for cash don't worry about paying salon prices. Simply go down to your local drug store and pick up a moisturizing hair mask for around $5.

What to do:

Apply the mask as directed on the package. Most will tell you to leave it on for 20 minutes and rinse. I suggest to pick up a shower cap with the product and start the treatment before bed and leave it in over night. It will not harm your hair to leave in longer than directed ensuring you are receiving the full effects of the product.

Top two causes for dry hair:

Over Shampooing: Most people think squeaky clean hair equals healthy hair. However, shampoos contain cleansing chemicals stripping your hair of the natural oils which keep it moisturized. Make sure to use proper amounts of product so you won't have to over shampoo to get them out.

Heat: Using curling irons/straighteners, blow dryers, hot curlers, and heat in general is a recipe for dry damaged hair.

Detanglers

This tip is to all my fellow long haired beauties. Please for the love of everything that's hairy, use a hair detangler. The time to break it out is when it's still difficult to brush through after using a conditioner. When you brush your hair in a hurry it's easy to rip through knots to get the job done. This WILL destroy your hair. The weaker strands of hair can break off causing a frizz look. Not pretty. This means more products to control it leaving your hair susceptible to drying out because of all the cleansers and shampoos you will have to use to get out extra products. Be kind to your hair.

What to do:

After you get out of the shower towel dry your hair. Then apply a detangler to your damp hair. Most leave-in conditioners also work well as a detangler. Grab your brush and start from the bottom of your beautiful locks and work your way through the knots to the top – one knot at a time.

Fly-Aways

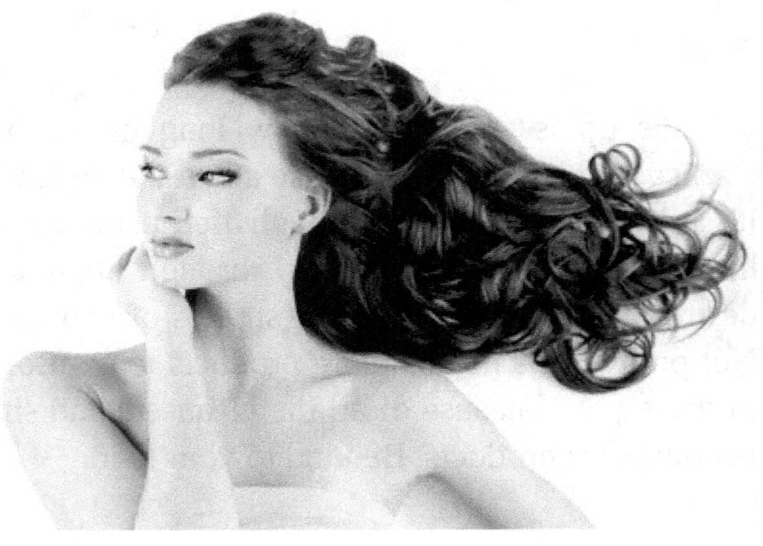

Since hair can get damaged from styling and highlights, fly-aways or broken strands of hair occur, sticking up when you want them to lay down. There are different tricks to keep them under control, mostly with the use of products to give you the perfect "hair color box" look.

1 One way to tame fly-aways is by using a glob of anti-frizz serum after you are done styling your hair. Smooth it evenly over the top of your hair, as well as the tips. This will weigh down some of the rogue hair but it doesn't eliminate all of them. You can find anti-frizz serum at any drug store.

2 My favorite frizz control technique is to spray a full bristled brush with hairspray and comb lightly over the problem area.

3 Another great solution is to use a hair molding cream or wax product. These types of products are usually heavier and can take on the job. If you use too much it can leave your hair looking dirty. Use lightly!

Hair Nutrition

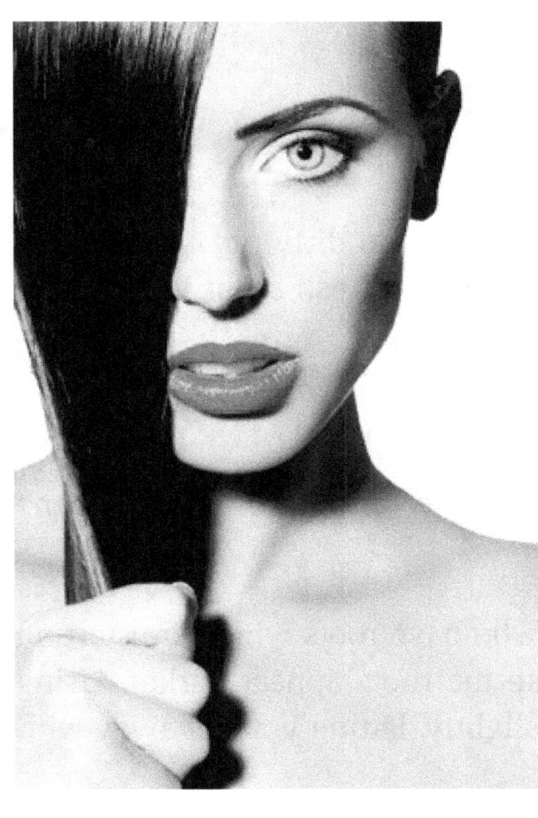

Diet, exercise, and nutrition can affect the vibrancy of your flowing hair. Exercising causes more blood flow which can aid in the delivery of additional nutrients and oxygen to your follicles for healthy, shiny hair. For the same reason, exercise will bring more nutrients to your skin cells for a glowing complexion.

Diet is the other hair health helper. Since your hair is 97% protein, low protein diets can take the robustness out of your locks. The most damaging aspect to beautiful hair can be rapid weight loss. It's been proven crash diets make hair fall out because of how it can stress the body. Lack of nutrition will also cause slow hair growth.

Dry Shampoo

Dry shampoo is hair's secret weapon. The solution to dirty or oily hair, dry shampoo acts as an absorbent, leaving hair with a fresh scent without the use of water.

When to use:

1 A great time to use dry shampoo is when you're on the go and you don't have time to wash your hair.

2 This powdery product is ideal for blondes who have roots which are starting to come in. Roots heavy with oil can make the roots appear darker. Using dry shampoo will lighten up the darker shades slightly, letting you get away with fewer trips to the salon.

3 The second and/or third day after you wash your hair is my favorite time for using this product to help in between washes. Washing your hair everyday will dry it out leaving it dull and damaged.

If you run out of dry shampoo, try baby powder in it's place.

Sectioning Guide To Curling & Straighting Hair

While sitting in "the chair" on photo shoots or commercials, hairstylists always have a plan when curling or straightening hair. If you begin the process without being organized, you could miss pieces leaving you susceptible to embarrassment. Always attack in sections.

Basic technique is important. However, there are different types of curls, waves, and volumizers which require different sets of skills. If you want a more polished curl to hold for a longer time, try using a curling iron smaller than an inch. After curling each strand section, pin the curl to your head allowing it to set and cool. If you are looking to add volume, I suggest to use a curling iron bigger than an inch and a half. For a sexy wave, curl and leave hairspray to handle the rest. This ensures the curl won't set too tight.

Although curling is time consuming and there is a larger margin for error, straightening can be just as involved. If you have thick hair you may have to generously use your flat iron.

How to section:

To start, your hair should to be fully dry. You will need a hair clip which will hold most of your hair at the same time. Choose a hair clip strong enough for the job.

Begin by gathering all your hair as if you were beginning a ponytail. Now, use your finger or the end of a comb to section off the bottom third of your hair.

Leave the bottom section hanging down and clip the top section up to keep it out of your way.

Divide the hair hanging down in half and drape equal amounts over each shoulder. You can begin using your curling or flat iron on those first pieces, which are the easiest sections to work with.

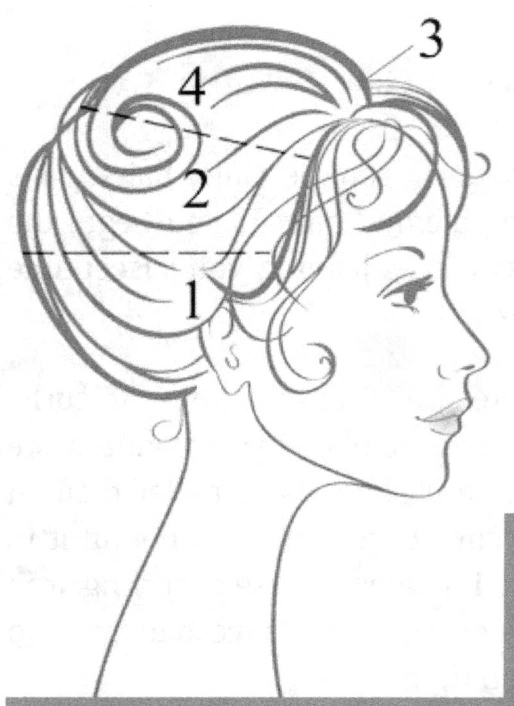

123 After working through the first section with your iron you will need to prepare the next sections you will work on.

4 Divide the remaining hair into thirds, working on the left and right sides, leaving the middle/top (similar to a mohawk) for last.

Matching Curls:

On set, a hair stylist instructed me how to get curls exactly the same on each side. He explained to curl one side using the iron in my right hand and on the opposite side use the curling iron in my left. That way the curls are going the same direction. I tried it and it worked!

Glamorize A Ponytail

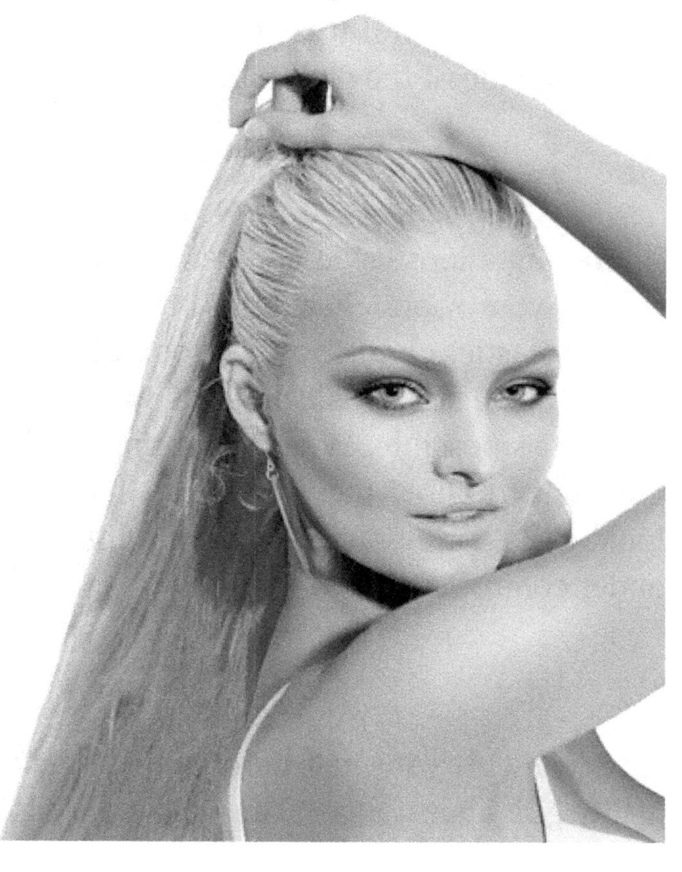

Ponytails are a great way to get your hair out of the way when you don't feel like dealing with it. While a ponytail is simple and uninspired, there are small things you can do to add spark giving you a more personal, styled look.

A small bouffant

This look is elegant, sleek, and can create a big impact with a small amount of work. First, comb through your hair brushing it back. Then create a small section about two inches wide and a ½ inch deep at the center front of your hair line. While holding the section, pull it towards your face and tease the underside. Next, create another section with the same dimensions directly behind the first and tease both sides. Now pull both sections back towards your crown. Grab a thick bristled brush to smooth over the top layer, lightly brushing it in the process. Keep in mind to be gentle and not brush out the tease. Next, twist the ends of the combined section one or two times, creating a rope like effect making it possible to pin a bobby pin to hold the hair together. After placing the bobby pin, you can create the ponytail using all your hair, including the teased top section. And voila, you just spiced up the plain ponytail! To make the bouffant bigger, take your finger and gently massage into the teased section to loosen it. If you want to make the bump smaller, try running your brush through it lightly.

Wrap strands around the hair elastic.

This one is an oldie but goody. Your mom probably did this to you as a kid.

After you've created your ponytail, take strands of your hair and wrap it around the hair elastic until it is concealed. Use a bobby pin to hold the hair in place on the underside of the ponytail.

The low side ponytail.

Having a loose side ponytail is sexy and trendy. You can even add volume by teasing your roots. Start by bringing all your hair over to one side and use your clip or elastic, giving you the look of a vixen. If you have time to curl, go for it. For an elegant look, sleek is the way to go. Use a flat iron to make your hair as smooth as possible. When you bring it all to one side, try not to make the elastic too tight to allow the ponytail to fall naturally. Since sleek is a more together look, make sure you finish with a light coat of hair spray to keep the fly-aways under control.

Curl it.

If you curl your hair before creating a ponytail, you will generate an ultimate girlie girl appearance. This can be charming while at the same time giving yourself volume.

The Messy Bun

 The messy bun look is stylish while practical. This look is fashionable, trendy, and can be used in casual and formal situations. Here is the best part: It's easy to do!

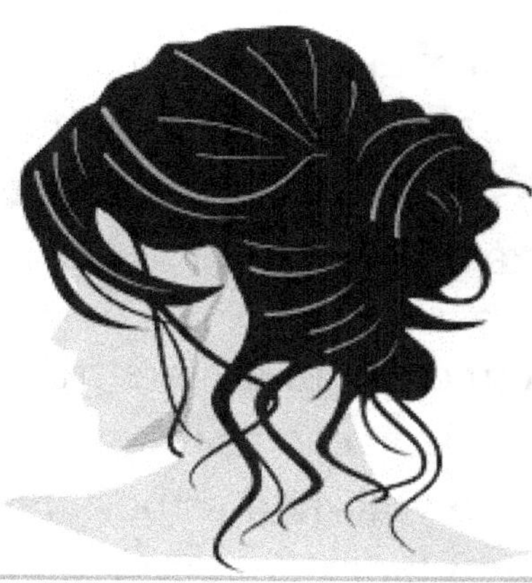

There are a lot of different hair types and different ways to execute the messy bun look depending on the length and thickness of your hair. In a situation where you want the look to last, I would suggest curling your hair first before you start twisting. This will give it more volume, thickness, and it's more likely to stay in place. My favorite way to wear it is low and to the side!

Pro Tips

Christina Cessna - Celebrity Hair Stylist

"My favorite hair secret is adding a shine/cellophane after having color done. Hair is then left with unbelievable shine which lasts twice as long."

"A good conditioning treatment mixed with a hair mask is another must for healthy looking hair. Go under the dryer, stream room or shower for a minimum of 10 minutes after applying the product then rinse. This will ensure the product goes to the cuticle of the hair for ultimate repair."

"When blow-drying hair, it is best to use a hair serum or oil to protect from heat as well as revive, strengthen, and condition the hair. You can also mix the product with a heat protectant to ensure as little damage to your hair as possible. When finished, run a tiny bit of serum on the ends of your hair taming possible frizz or fly-aways. To avoid an oily look, try to keep the serum away from the roots."

Rachel Cannon - Actress
Two and a Half Men

"Since I have wavy hair, which has a mind of it's own, I have learned the best way to keep it under control by using product!! I love mixing a leave-in conditioner and curl creme (like the one from bumble and bumble) when I first get out of the shower. This allows me to comb my fingers through my hair, since I don't use a hairbrush."

"To diffuse my hair, I'll add a few more products as it begins to dry. First, I'll add a light mouse then let my hair dry a bit. Next, I'll add a wax pomade followed by more dry time. Last, a light hairspray helps hold my golden mane together. My hair then stays in check all day, full of attitude which puts me where I need to be for all of my auditions or meetings."

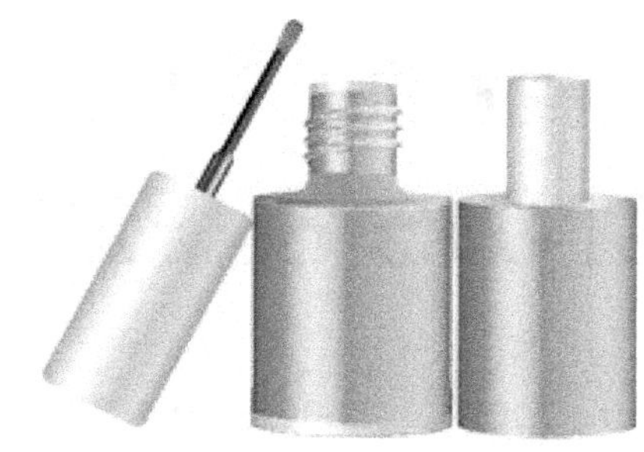

Chapter Four: HANDS & FEET

It's unlikely you will flip open a magazine and see a model with poorly manicured nails. Probably because callused feet and unkempt nails are not very pleasant to look at -- ultimately distracting from the advertisement. Taking care of your extremities will make you appear put-together. It can also give you a very feminine feeling which will add to your overall attractiveness. Moisturizer and mani/pedi's can go a long way and they should be on every girls regular to-do lists.

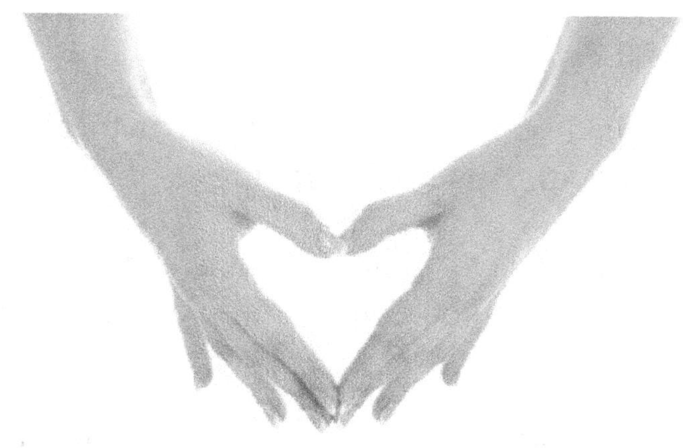

Nails

Simple sheer pinks or nude colors are a perfect natural way to display your hands and feet. Whether you are working or going about your daily activities, having a manicured look gives a great impression and lets people know you take care of yourself. You never know who is watching, like a future employer, which is motivation to maintain a polished look.

It's not always affordable to make a regular trip to the nail salon and some of us don't have the time. Here are a few tips on self-manicures as well as some advice on how to manage your nails in between salon visits.

Nail Tips

Always have nail polish on hand for a quick coat to give your nails strength. This will help prevent your nails from chipping as often.

Carry a nail file. It's always great to have a nail file nearby in case of emergencies or if your bored you can clean up and even out your nails to pass the time.

When doing house work or gardening, wear rubber gloves. This will help keep your nails clean and help prevent breakage. Chemicals can also cause dryness, which in turn could make your nails brittle and unappealing.

Apply hand moisturizer as often as possible. Try having your favorite moisturizer near you when you watch TV, and next to your hand soap in the bathroom or kitchen. Moisturizing will not only make your hands soft but can also help strengthen your nails.

Keep your nails at a manageable length. I love long nails but I know my clumsiness would never allow me to have them for a long period of time. I keep my nails short so they are always even and beautiful.

Try to file your nails in a shape which mirrors the curve of your nail base.

When applying nail polish, don't shake the bottle, as this will create air bubbles. Try rolling the bottle back and forth between your hands.

Before applying nail polish, wipe your nails with nail polish remover to remove natural oils and any residues so your nail polish won't peel as easily.

When painting your nails, start with a base coat to strengthen and protect. Then finish your polish with a clear top coat to add shine.

Healthy Diet = Happy Nails.

Standing on your feet all day in heels is a treacherous task. The pain of high heels not only gives you aching feet but an aching lower back as well. Models know this feeling all too well because the shoes worn in photos or on the runway aren't always the right size – ouch! Let's not forget the awful things our feet go through in normal daily lives and exercise routines. Because our feet carry us every day, we should appreciate them and give them extra care.

Foot Care

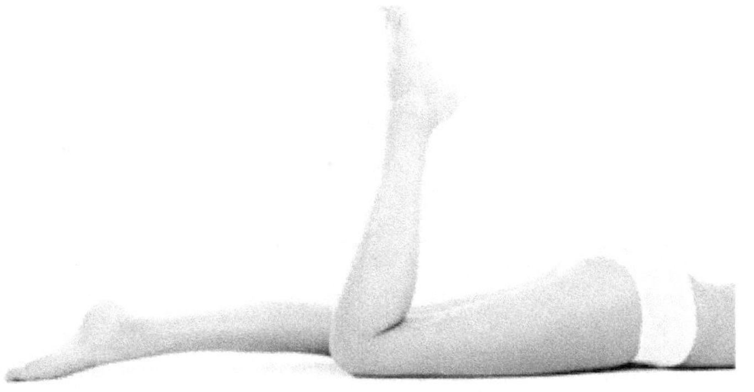

Taking care of your feet isn't only relaxing but it can make you more beautiful. Cracked, peeling feet are unattractive to look at and many times can be very painful.

Rough Feet – If your feet are rough and callused, using a pumice stone is a great way to rub off the hard skin. If you have never tried this method before be careful not to take off too much or it could be sore.

Soften Your Feet – At night, take a bath or soak your feet in warm water. Then coat your feet in a heavy foot cream (Vaseline or petroleum jelly works well too). After throw on a pair of heavy socks and hop into bed. When you wake up in the morning your feet will feel soft and moisturized.

Honey Foot Soak

For those really long days, a foot soak is worth the small amount of effort. Grab a foot soak tub and make this honey concoction.

1 tbs honey
1 tbs liquid Soap (dish soap works)
1 tsp vanilla extract
2 tbs almond oil

Fill the tub with warm water. Add the mixture and soak for about 10 minutes. Since honey is a natural anti-bacterial, anti-viral, and anti-fungal antioxidant it serves as a perfect ingredient. Raw honey has even been known to cure athlete's foot.

Pro Tips

Amanda Lockwood - Model/Actress/Twin Sister

"When I'm on the go and don't have time to give myself a proper manicure, I give myself what I call, "my 2 minute manicure." I quickly file my nails evenly then use nail polish remover to wipe off old polish residue and natural oils. Last, I add a few coats of clear nail polish! When your in a hurry, clear nail polish is perfect because it's fast drying and if you happen to smudge...it's invisible! It's quick and easy making it a sneaky way to pull off a freshly manicured look."

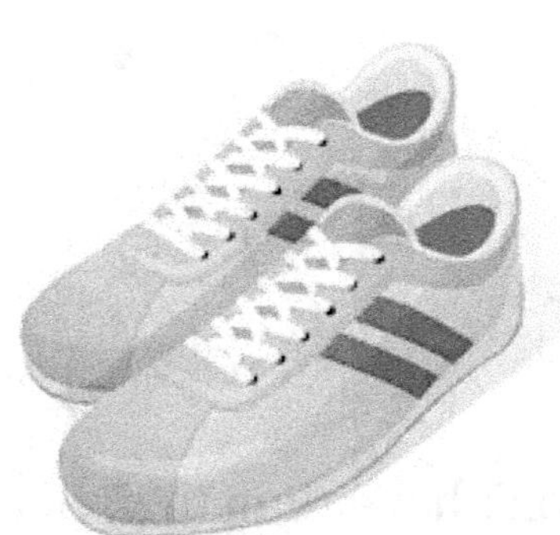

Chapter Five: FITNESS

The greatest argument for being fit and exercising regularly is longevity. If it's not convincing enough, regular exercise fights depression, heart disease, diabetes, hypertension, stroke, and aids in cognitive function. However this is a book on beauty. Let's talk about the cosmetic effects of staying fit.

The beauty benefits are so great when it comes to your skin, hair, and toning you can't look your absolute best without routinely hitting the gym, going for a long hike, or participating in any other form of exercise.

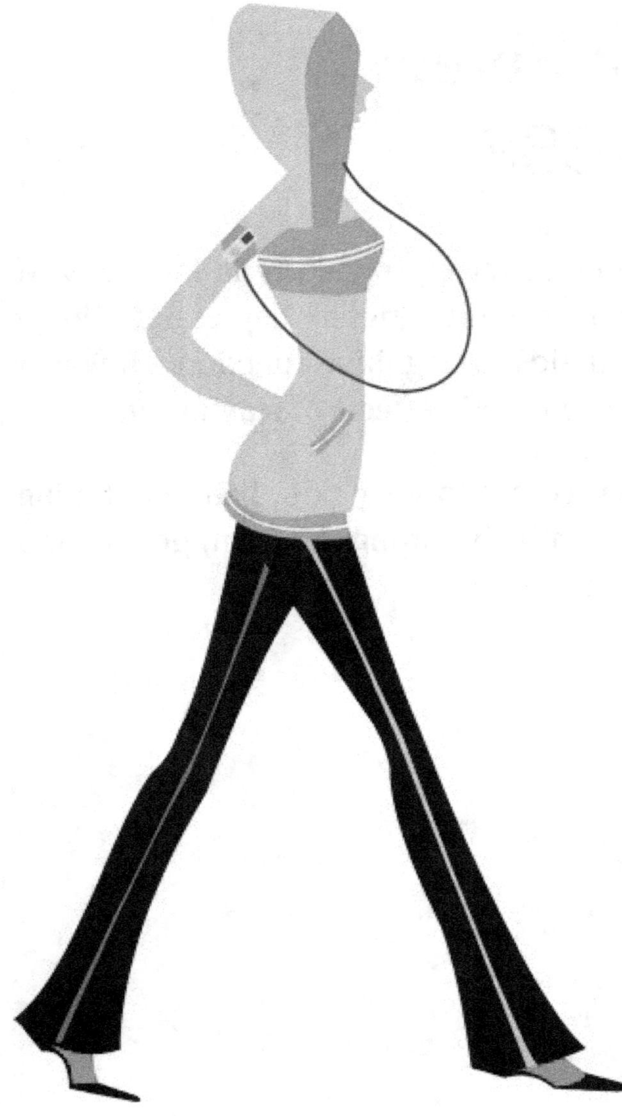

Skin

Increasing circulation from exercise activity will deliver oxygen and nutrients to your body at high performance, you'll notice glowing skin after a work out. The extra boost can infuse skin cells with oxygen, helping collagen production and plumping skin cells. This means you can fight signs of aging and get rosy cheeks in the process!

Weight Reducer

Some benefits of routine workouts are toning, better posture, weight loss, and balance. These results are ideal for anyone looking to better their physique. Being active will burn the extra calories your body may not use if it were inactive, instead of storing them as fat.

Acne & Hair

Exercise isn't an acne solution but it can help control breakouts. Doctor's say exercise mediates the production of testosterone related hormones (DHEA & DHT) -- the horrid chemicals related to acne. Sweating even helps with acne because it unclogs pores.

STRESS RELIEVER

he extra blood and oxygen your heart pumps from exercise nourish brain cells making them more active. This extra activity elevates natural serotonin production (the chemical which makes you happy and content). It also stimulates your endorphins (the feel good chemical from the brain – giving you an overall feeling of euphoria) equaling less stress, anxiety, and depression. A good work out can alleviate the daily pressures and hardships you might face in everyday life.

Forget the myth about women about women who use weights will look like a body builder; we don't have enough testosterone. Weights can actually break up pockets of cellulite by firming your muscles which can push the fat up and out. Not only will using weights redefine your muscles to work more efficiently but with the right diet and work out regimen you can sculpt your muscles into a work of art.

"Physical fitness is not only one of the most important keys to a healthy body, it is the basis of dynamic and creative intellectual activity."

- JFK

"I still need more healthy rest in order to work at my best. My health is the main capital I have and I want to administer it intelligently."

- Ernest Hemingway

"Leave all the afternoon for exercise and recreation, which are as necessary as reading. I will rather say more necessary because health is worth more than learning."

- Thomas Jefferson

"The only way to keep your health is to eat what you don't want, drink what you don't like, and do what you'd rather not."

- Mark Twain

"Every human being is the author of his own health or disease."

- Budda

Pro Tips

Khalid Benmbarek – Personal Trainer

"My clients have seen dramatic transformations in their bodies, minds and spirits when I combine a dynamic combination of interval training, plyometrics, cross fit, circuit training, resistance/strength training, speed training, boxing and cardio-vascular training, stairs, and stretching. A combination of proven techniques in an intense yet fun atmosphere have given my clients the bodies they have always dreamed of."

Sara Bronson - Model/Actress
Former Deal or No Deal Model

"For my diet and workout regimen - I love my *Clean Eating* and *Shape* magazines! *Clean Eating* has great, recipes made from real, whole foods and *Shape* is great when I need to switch up my workout. I rely on my magazines for fitness and diet motivation!!"

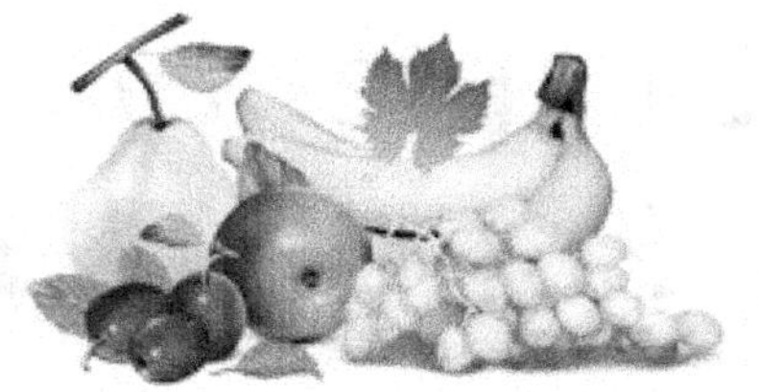

Chapter Six:
DIET & NUTRITION

The best epiphany I've ever had was acceptance. We all love to eat fast food, cookies, and cakes. But I know as a model this cannot be part of a healthy meal plan. Evil temptations such as sugar loaded treats, foods high in trans fats, and unhealthy heart fats are a test to all of our will power.

The first thing to start a diet should began with a routine at the grocery store. Make sure to never have junk food readily available in your cupboards by never buying it. Chips, soda, and other sugary goodies are out of reach for good reason. We're not made of steel.

When it comes to vitamins, make the habit of taking omega 3's and multivitamins at the same time everyday after a meal. Ensuring you are giving your body the extra love it deserves. You only have one life and one body. Treating it well and putting good things into it will in turn give you a better quality of life. Healthy living can translate into confidence because you are doing something for yourself everyday. Let's not forget the other wonderful positive side effects: preventing cancer, glowing skin, a thin figure, healthy skin/hair, and self-esteem.

Green Tea

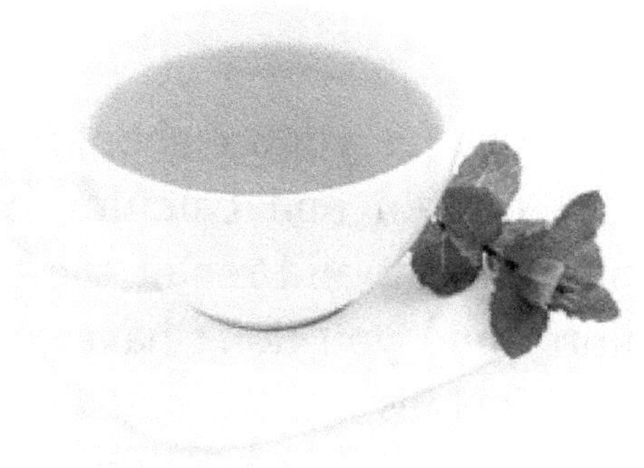

Green tea has many benefits which aid in beauty and health. While recommended daily consumption is debated, drinking four to five cups a day seems to be the average suggested amount. Of course, consult your doctor about what daily dose is right for you.

Green tea aids in weight loss because it contains catechins. Catechins is a chemical which lowers cholesterol and burns calories reducing your overall body fat. It's also good for your teeth because it prevents plaque from being formed by inhibiting bacteria growth.

If used as a topical treatment green tea can prevent UVB skin disorders like photo-aging and melanoma. The wonder tonic can also help acne and has been proven to be just as effective as benzoyl peroxide. Sweet!

prevents plaque   antioxidant   weight loss stimulator   helps immune system   lowers cholesterol   fights cancer   burns calories/calorie free improves cardiovascular health   protects skin

Low Fat Yogurt

Low fat yogurt should be in your beauty diet because it contains tons of protein and calcium, which can fight hunger, stimulate weight loss by burning fat, and repair the body. It's a great on-the-go snack when you're in a hurry and you don't have to feel guilty eating it. Usually, calcium and mineral deficiencies are the cause of dry hair and brittle nails, along with dehydration. Grabbing a yogurt will ensure you are not lacking anything your body needs for the day. The calcium stimulates hair growth and makes it shiny, as well as making your nails strong.

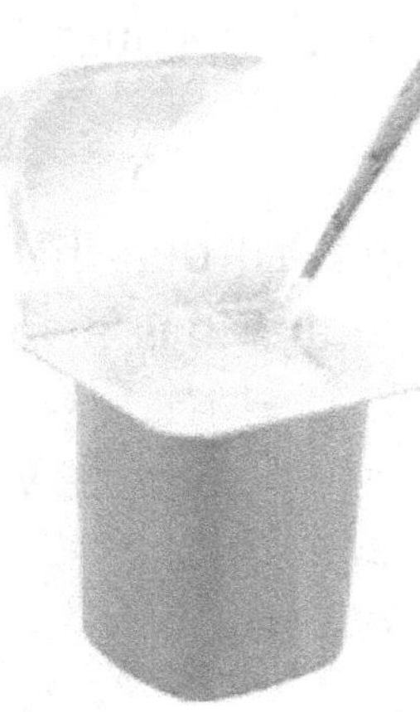

Yogurt is made from milk by adding cultures which transforms the milk's sugar and lactose into lactic acid. The cultures added have good bacteria in it which contain live microorganisms which help with digestion and can kill bad bacteria. The low fat, low calorie immune system booster also contains an anti-carcinogenic – which means it fights cavities too!

Considered an essential fatty acid, omega-3s play a major role in beauty, body, and brain function. Your body needs fatty acids to be healthy. However, *researchers have said omega-3 fatty acids are the only nutrient your body cannot reproduce. We have to find it elsewhere. You can take a supplement of omega-3s in the form of a fish oil capsule or eat omega rich foods like some cold water fish such as salmon, halibut and mackerel. Some of the other foods you can find omega-3's include walnuts, spinach, flax, soybeans, and whole grains.

Not only are omega-3s your health's best friend, the beauty benefits are astounding. It's been proven it will improve skin condition and make it glow. Fatty acids help hold in moisture and replenish lipids which is what keeps our skin flexible. Taken over a long period of time omega-3s can even reverse the effects of sun damage and photo-aging. Other beauty bonuses are luxurious hair and stronger nails. I noticed a major difference about a month after I started taking the capsules. I've received the most compliments on my hair and skin AFTER I'd been taking the fish oil supplements!

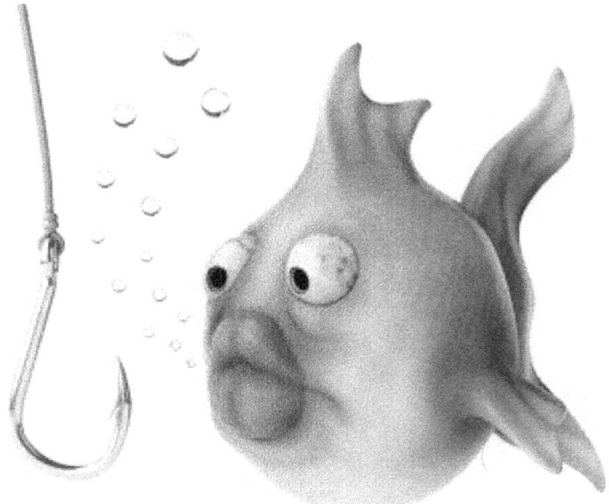

Now, we know omega-3s give us beautiful hair, glowing skin and strong nails. You can also take omega-3s due to all this other additional interesting research. We should also know our bodies need a tremendous amount of the omega-3 fatty acids to function. Why? Because the human brain is comprised of 60% fats, and approximately half of the fat is DHA omega-3. Meaning the organ which controls all of our body systems is a big piece of fat! Having fatty deficiencies in our brain have been linked to Alzheimer's disease, mood disorders, anxiety, depression, bi-polar disorder, and other mood altering catastrophes millions of people suffer from.

Keeping our brain sharp is just one of its health miracles. The biggest and best benefit of taking omega-3s is what it does for our heart health. By making platelets in the blood less sticky it will prevent clotting, which can reduce blood pressure and heart disease. It also reduces triglyceride levels, which are fat deposits in our blood. High levels of triglycerides and cholesterol increase your chances of heart complications.

Omega-3s are good in many ways, but as a woman, I'm mentioning it for a specific reason: omega-3s reduce inflammation helping with our menstruation cycle. Fish oil has been known to stabilize moods during the time of the month and reduces cramps. Since inflammation is one of the reasons women feel a dull pain before and during a cycle, taking a omega-3 supplement is a natural remedy with a ton of benefits.

*Research found on http://www.webmd.com

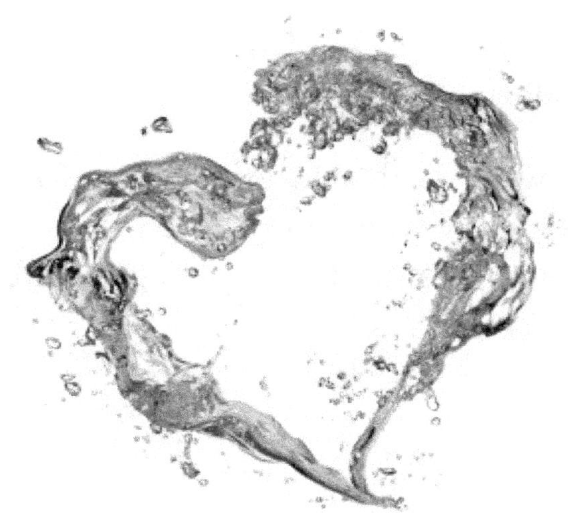

Water

Have you ever noticed your skin not glowing and you see bags under your eyes? When you look tired and feel sluggish it may be caused from dehydration. Everyone needs energy to work long days, making water the the most important thing to keep you energetic, healthy, supple, and beautiful. Our bodies are 70% water, therefore it's essential to all our important functional systems. Water aids organs like the liver and kidneys in ridding toxins and flushing infections out of our immune system. Being dehydrated not only makes us feel run down it takes out the suppleness in our skin cells which makes us appear healthy.

Beautiful looking skin, nails, and hair can all be attributed to H20. Dehydration will make wrinkles appear deeper than they really are, cause our nails to break and discolor, and our hair to be dull, dry and brittle. Since water flushes out toxins and impurities, our skin will appear fresh, clear, and moisturized. Water also stimulates growth in our hair (which is 12-15% water) by transporting amino acids, vitamins, and minerals to hair follicles.

Drinking water is also a fantastic tool for losing weight. If you drink a glass of water before and after every meal you will feel fuller, reducing the likelihood of over eating. The best part: it's zero calories! If you switch soda, coffee, and fruit juices to water your caloric intake will be reduced drastically, making it far easier to lose weight.

To ensure you drink enough water:

1 Carry a bottle of water with you everywhere (preferably nalgene or steel bottles). You never know when you will be stuck somewhere like a grocery store, traffic jam, gym, or the airport. Try getting something cute to drink out of.

2 Make sure to drink a glass when you wake up, before coffee, and before bed.

3 Drink a full glass before meals.

4 Keep a glass of water at your desk to drink from regularly.

5 Add lemon for more excitement.

6 Never enter the gym or workout location without a full bottle (you should have at least one bottle of water for every half hour of exercise).

7 Keep an empty glass/cup next to your water filter. When you pass by, fill it up and chug.

8 Have a cup in your house you can call "my big cup." Always know where it is and always make sure it's full.

Have you ever felt hungry an hour after your post workout snack? Your brain could be telling you you're hungry, confusing hunger with with dehydration. You should hydrate before and after your workouts to tame those false hunger pains.

Antioxidants, Vitamins & Free Radicals

Aging is a woman's worst enemy. Side effects from aging, such as fine lines, wrinkles, and sun damage can take away adolescent allure. Planning a full attack to slow down the normal process of oxidation (the damage to our cells to make us appear older) is something to think about. Oxidation can be accelerated by pollution, sunlight, alcohol, and smoking. Sunblock and a healthy lifestyle is the beginning to maintaining youthful beauty, while antioxidants and vitamins will help with the rest.

Damaged cells called free radicals are oxidized unstable atoms. Damaged atoms try to repair themselves by taking electrons from their surroundings or the healthy stuff from other cells. Antioxidants can be offered as a treatment since they are chemicals which offer their own electrons, thus sparing your healthy cells from damage. Antioxidants = oxidized-atom crime fighter.

*Researchers say antioxidants are helpful because they can reduce the look of fine lines and wrinkles, improve the look of skin, and protect us from further sun damage. People who study their benefits also say you have to keep a continual supply of antioxidants because once the antioxidant looses its electron it ceases to be useful. Therefore, you should take vitamins with antioxidants in them and eat antioxidant rich foods everyday. Some vitamin and antioxidant treatments can work from the outside in. Nutrition and diets can work from the inside out, targeting harmful free radicals and sun damage.

There are multiple ways to get antioxidants, omega-3s, and vitamins daily. Drink green tea as much as possible because of the richness of its antioxidants. Take a multivitamin and omega-3 supplement everyday with a meal to ensure the vitamins have something to absorb with while the body is processing it. Eat vitamin and antioxidant rich foods like blueberries, spinach, tomatoes, walnuts, almonds, peaches, and avocados. Topically (applied to skin), make sure your face and body lotions contain skin and anti-age protecting awesomeness too. Try to look for facial moisturizers which contain green tea extract.

Vitamin A: This antioxidant helps your

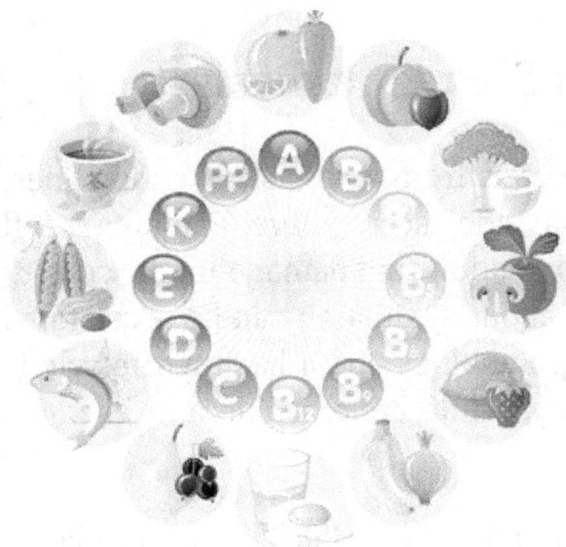

skin maintain moisture and restores elastic fibers which keeps the skin taut, ultimately helping anti-aging effects like fine wrinkles, sunspots, and rough skin. Vitamin A is best in a concentrated gel or cream form.

Vitamin B: Essential for all our body's cells. B Vitamins can boost the rate of your metabolism as well as your immune and nervous systems. Deficiencies can also lead to dry and itchy skin.

Vitamin C: This vitamin is known to help protect skin from sun damage and cancer. It's also great for boosting your immune system which will in turn speed up your skin repairing system, making it an antioxidant vitamin powerhouse. Vitamin C is also important in the formation of collagen to hold skin cells together and other body tissues.

Vitamin D: Vitamin D helps your body consume calcium which is good for your bones and teeth. It also helps regulate cells, systems, and organs throughout the body. One way to get vitamin D is by having your body create it after it reacts to ultraviolet light or sunlight.

Vitamin E: A fat-soluble vitamin found in many foods, fats, and oils. Vitamin E is an antioxidant superhero which fights off free radicals.

Flavoniods: Found in green tea and even chocolate. Flavoniods can protect from inflammation and cancer. It also protects adverse effects of sunlight exposure.

Vitamin K: Another fat-soluble vitamin which aids in reducing bruising and broken capillaries by helping with the coagulation of blood. I started to use a vitamin K gel under my eyes for dark circles and I saw results within a week.

*Research found on http://www.webmd.com

Sugar

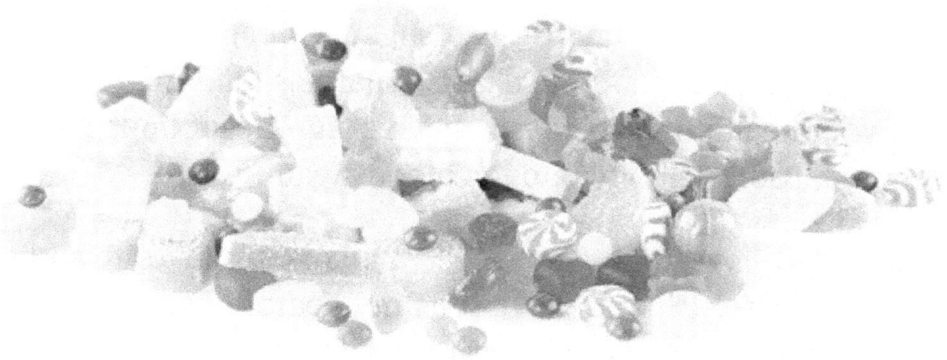

Have you ever looked at the ingredient labels on the food in your cupboard? Almost everything contains chemicals, lots of sugar, or high fructose corn syrup. The best way to stay lean is to accept the fact sugar and processed foods are empty calories which make you gain weight. It's bad for your skin and bad for your teeth. Instead, change your eating habits to fresh foods, devoid of high fructose corn syrup, and contain no unwanted chemicals.

I know Cheetos are tasty, soda is delicious, and Oreo's are to die for, but at what cost? Gaining weight and not being comfortable with the way you look? Your health? I had to give up all those things a long time ago after I realized it would help my career by making me more competitive. The second I gave up sodas, I noticed less fat in my body a week later. When I moved onto fresher foods, I noticed my energy levels were higher. I took sugar out of my diet completely and switched over my sweeteners to natural sweetener replacements (like agave nectar), making maintaining a thin weight a breeze. I never looked back.

Bad sugar really is the devil and you can't get away from it unless you make an effort. It's even addictive, which will have you coming back again and again. Toughen up and realize your overall health is much more important than a tub of ice cream. Looking better in clothes will give you priceless confidence in life. It worked for me.

Anti-Sugar Helpful Tips:

Replace artificial sweeteners and refined sugar with agave nectar. Agave nectar comes from cactus and is rich in nutrients, vitamins, and minerals which can be beneficial to your health. It also doesn't have a significant impact on blood-sugar levels because it absorbs slowly into the bloodstream.

Grab low fat yogurt instead of ice cream. Vanilla is my favorite and satisfies my sweet tooth every time. I like to have it as my "before bedtime, watching TV, I wish I had something sweet" snack. Watch out for fruit added yogurts. Add your own fresh fruit since many have sugary syrup added.

Have trail mix on hand and ditch the cookies. Trail mix is a great for an in-between-meal snack. It's healthy and will hold you over until it's meal time. The best trail mix contain whole nuts, uncovered raisins and dates. Be aware of coated raisins with palm oil covering because it's full of saturated fats.

Don't buy anything that will tempt you. IIf it's not there you won't eat it. I'm personally too lazy to go to the store just for cookies.

Keep healthy snacks in the fridge and cupboards at eye level. Cut up veggies and fruits like carrots and apples are perfect to have at your eyeline. If you must have sugary temptations around for guests or leftovers from a party, store them in a far place where it will take effort to get to them. Maybe you'll think twice on the far walk to the basement.

Read ingredient labels. Generally, the shorter the ingredient list the healthier. Know what the ingredients are and their benefits. Lots of companies like to reword chemicals and sugars to trick us into thinking it's something else rather than sugar. The simpler the better. If I have a tough choice between two products, the one with the shortest chemical list wins my decision.

Fruit, fruit, fruit - Fruit has natural fructose making it sweet, good for you, contains lots of antioxidants and you can eat tons of it. You'll never have to worry about going in for a second helping.

No more soda - ever! Trade soda for water, it's zero calories, it hydrates you (giving you energy), it flushes out toxins, and makes your skin look beautiful. To make it more exciting, add cucumber or lemon and pretend you're at a day spa.

If you must drink alcohol, have a vodka and club soda, then add lime for some flavor. Darker alcohols will make you hung over because they contain a higher concentration of congeners (the chemical which causes hangover symptoms); and sugary fruit drinks have tons of calories and make you crave even more sweet stuff.

Accept reality. You can't have king size candy bars and cookies to snack on daily. You have to make sacrifices if you want to change.

Pro Tips

Patricia Kara - Model/Host/Actress
Currently Spoke's Person/Model for NBC's Deal or No Deal

"Eat consistently throughout the day, smaller portions. Don't deprive yourself of your favorites, just don't overindulge. There are many healthy and yummy snacks as alternatives. One of my favorites is FAGE Greek yogurt with Honey or sugar free Maple Syrup and cinammon. Sometimes I add raw oatmeal, Ground flax and bran cereal to the yogurt. If its a warm day and your in the mood for a frozen treat, mix some chopped up fresh fruit with the yogurt and chill in freezer for an hour... scoop like ice cream. ENJOY!!!"

Laura Mutter - Celebrity Nutrition Consultant

"**Vitamin C**: Vitamin C helps in the build up of collagen, which reduces wrinkles. When your skin has more collagen your skin retains its elasticity and wrinkles take longer to form. Kiwi fruit is the best source of vitamin C. Other good sources are oranges, mango, honeydew and papaya."